CARDIO STRENGTH TRAINING

Rodale books may be purchased for business or promotional use or for special sales. For information, please write to: Special Markets Department, Rodale Inc., 733 Third Avenue, New York, NY 10017

Printed in the United States of America
Rodale Inc. makes every effort to use acid-free ♾, recycled paper ♲.

Photographs by Mitch Mandel/Rodale Images
Book design by Christopher Rhoads

Library of Congress Cataloging-in-Publication Data

Dos Remedios, Robert.
    Cardio strength training : torch fat, build muscle, and get stronger faster / by Robert dos Remedios.
        p.   cm.
    Includes index.
    ISBN-13 978–1–60529–655–5 paperback
    1. Physical fitness.   2. Exercise.   I. Title.
RA781.D586   2009
613.7—dc22   2009042723

Distributed to the trade by Macmillan

4   6   8   10   9   7   5   3   paperback original

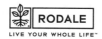

LIVE YOUR WHOLE LIFE™

We inspire and enable people to improve their lives and the world around them
For more of our products visit **rodalestore.com** or call 800-848-4735

CARDIO STRENGTH TRAINING

TORCH FAT, BUILD MUSCLE, AND GET STRONGER FASTER

Robert dos Remedios, cscs

RODALE

To my wife Francine and my daughter Annabella—I LOVE YOU!
To all of my mentors and friends in this industry and to all of my athletes,
both past and present, THANK YOU! You have all helped to shape
and mold me into the coach that I am today.

CONTENTS

FOREWORD.. viii

INTRODUCTION x

Chapter 1: What Is Cardio Strength Training? 1

Chapter 2: The Science behind Cardio Strength Training 5

Chapter 3: Cardio Strength Training Modes.. 9

Chapter 4: Getting Your Body Ready for Cardio Strength Training 13

Chapter 5: Complexes 41

Chapter 6: Timed Sets 107

Chapter 7: Tabata Protocol 191

Chapter 8: The Great Outdoors 201

Chapter 9: More Tools for Our Cardio Strength Training Toolbox 207

Chapter 10: High-Powered Nutrition 219

APPENDIX 225

INDEX 236

FOREWORD

"... in an information-rich world, the wealth of information means a dearth of something else: a scarcity of whatever it is that information consumes. What information consumes is rather obvious: It consumes the attention of its recipients. Hence, a wealth of information creates a poverty of attention and a need to allocate that attention efficiently among the overabundance of information sources that might consume it."

—HERBERT SIMON

We truly live in the information age. A simple Google search for a term that was relatively unknown 10 years ago—for example "Brazilian jiu jitsu" can return over one million Web pages devoted to the topic. With the rapid growth of information, one can imagine that this number will double in less time than it's taken to reach this level.

Quite simply, there is more information on any topic available today than ever before—in fact, more information than you can possibly consume in a lifetime devoted to study. It's just growing that fast.

The problem today is not a lack of information—it's a lack of filtering that information. So how do you filter information? At this point, there is so much information available that you *need* to filter out just as much as you retain.

My personal filter is to heavily prioritize information that comes from "real-world" practitioners whose livelihood depends upon delivering results or solving problems (and I'm a fanatic for proof).

It's that simple. I put my faith in real-world results. And that's why I put my faith in Robert dos Remedios.

With a proven track record, Coach Dos has more subjects come through his laboratory (the weight room and the field), giving him more real-world information than you can find almost anywhere.

Dos is an expert at what he does—not because he is a high-profile coach that high-level athletic talents seek out to help refine their already considerable skills—but because he works with real people in the real world hundreds of times every single day.

The topic of cardio strength training is as cutting edge as it gets. It's now proven in the clinical realm that strength training or interval training both outperform aerobic training for conditioning and fat loss.

It's something that great coaches have known for years. They had to. Their job, their team's record, and their kids' futures and scholarships depended on it.

What science hasn't proven yet is that a strength training–interval training hybrid outperforms both strength and interval training when practiced independently.

It's something that Coach Dos knows. He has to.

Welcome to Dos's World. Wait for the researchers to catch up. . . .

—ALWYN COSGROVE

INTRODUCTION

My first book, *Men's Health Power Training*, was truly an amazing experience. The success of the book, the interest that it has generated, and, more importantly, all the success stories I have received have been the real blessing of that book. As people read it and took their training and fitness to another level, I started thinking, "Where do we go from here?" Wwas there anything more I could write about that would fit in nicely with the MHPT philosophy, perhaps another training modality that would be as effective as the lifting programs in the first book? The first thing that came to my mind when thinking of a natural follow-up book was "metabolic conditioning." I have received quite a bit of feedback and interest in the cardio strength training chapter in *Power Training*. This chapter basically covered non-traditional forms of cardio to promote fitness and conditioning while helping to shed fat. I began to think that I barely scratched the surface of this topic in this short chapter and that it would be a great topic for an entire training book.

Folks were becoming very intrigued with this type of training and how effective it really was. Now don't get me wrong, this type of interval-style cardio is not for the weak of heart (or body) or the average Joe or Jane who thinks that 30 minutes on the elliptical trainer while talking on their cell phone is "butt-kicking cardio." This type of training is TOUGH . . . very tough. Let's go back to the general foundation of MHPT: the overload principle. Simply put, you need to push yourself harder and harder in order to continue to see gains. From a metabolic conditioning standpoint, this principle is KING. If the work interval is short, the intensity needs to be very, very hard. As the duration of the intervals gets longer, there will be a natural decrease in intensity. All this will be explained in detail as we continue through the book, but just remember that "cardio strength training" will most likely be the most difficult form of cardio you will ever encounter. Trust me though, this hard work will pay off big time in fitness gains and fat loss. You will see changes in your body you would have never imagined.

Walk into any gym in America and you will see lines and lines of treadmills, stair climbers, and elliptical machines on which people are doing some form of steady state aerobic training. You know the type of exercise I'm talking about—somewhat easy, low intensity. These people might be having conversations with a neighbor, watching a television show, or even reading a book. This is NOT the type of metabolic training I will be covering in this book. From a fat loss and fitness standpoint, the training described above is completely inferior to cardio strength training. I will be highlighting, teaching, and persuading you buy into interval style training. This type of training is highlighted by short sessions of intermittent high intensity work. Let's just say you will be too busy to have that cell phone conversation if you are doing this type of training. In fact, you most likely wouldn't be able to dial correctly if you tried.

One of the most popular forms of what I call cardio strength training is the Tabata Protocol. Do a simple Google or Yahoo Internet search on this topic and you will see just how popular it is. A study published in 1996 in *Medicine and Science in Sports and Exercise* showed that this simple 4-minute protocol using negative rest periods (20 seconds of high intensity work followed by 10 seconds of rest) five times a week (a total of 20 minutes) was more effective than traditional steady state cardio performed for 60 minutes, five times per week. Yes, in a fraction of the time, they found greater aerobic and anaerobic gains in the short, high intensity interval group! The research is pretty astounding in proving the effectiveness of interval training and also often in proving the ineffectiveness of traditional cardio like running on treadmills and such. This shows again and again that the most effective and

Cardio for fat loss is all about creating a metabolic "disturbance" which forces the body to use energy to recover. Unfortunately, the form of cardio that you see being performed at most gyms nationwide (i.e. low-intensity treadmill or stationary bike work) does very little to create the kind of disturbance necessary for recovery metabolism. With metabolic resistance training, however, you are able to take intensity to a whole new level beyond what is possible with typical forms of cardio training. This equates to the greatest energy burn, and subsequently, unparalleled fat loss.

Joel Marion, CISSN, NSCA-CPT
Owner, Joel Marion Fitness Solutions

efficient form of cardio is some form of interval style training when compared to the old standard of spending long periods of time performing steady state exercise. To top it off, one of the major benefits of cardio strength training is the fact that you can get all of these amazing fitness gains and fat burning furnace-like effects without sacrificing your lean body mass; this is pretty darn important for most anyone who takes pride in their weight training and their muscle mass.

I am confident that this journey into the world of cardio strength training will be enlightening, effective, and often character building. It will change the way you view metabolic training and will hook you for life. As I said previously, this journey will not be easy and it will take work. It will, however, be well worth the effort. So why write this book? Why now? It's simple, just as I shared in *Men's Health Power Training*, I'm tired of seeing people do the wrong things in the gym—tired of seeing people not reach their fitness goals and become frustrated with the conditioning process. It's time to introduce you to the most effective and efficient form of cardio on the planet. Hold onto your seats folks; this is going to be a life-changing program for you!

WHAT IS CARDIO STRENGTH TRAINING?

You walk into the gym and you see lines of cardio machines—people exercising while talking on cell phones, watching television, or even having conversations with neighbors, all the while making sure to stay in their "fat-burning zones." Then you notice a guy tucked away in the corner of the gym, headphones on, huffing and puffing and sweating to the point of exhaustion. He's doing burpees, then he's doing squat jumps, then he's swinging a kettlebell. There seems to be no rhyme or reason to this maniac's exercise method: All you know is that it looks intense, a bit odd, and far from traditional. You can't look away; what the heck is going on there?

Well, this guy in the corner was doing a form of what I call cardio strength training—training highlighted by intense bouts of exercise and short rest periods. The question that begs to be asked is why so many of these "fat burners" on the cardio machines

are still carrying excess fat while this guy in the corner most likely looks lean, strong, and athletic. Well, first of all, this individual definitely had a plan in his choice of exercise. His goals were simple: get the most bang for his buck with these intervals and create the ever important "afterburn" effect in his metabolism that will serve as a calorie-burning furnace for hours and hours following his session. He also gets all these benefits in a fraction of the time these "fat burners" spend on their cardio machines. Too good to be true? Well, not exactly. As I tell the athletes I train every day, "There is a price to pay for success." In other words, don't confuse "short" with "easy."

Okay, so I have used the term "fat burners" a few times already, and I will admit I use it facetiously. The whole concept of exercising at lower intensities in order to maximize the amount of fat that you burn, rather than sugar or carbohydrate, is one of the great exercise

For years the idea of fat loss and resistance to fatigue has been directly linked to steady-state cardiovascular activity, however, there are much more efficient and fun ways to reach these goals. Some of the greatest tools that can be used for these goals are interval training and kettlebell complexes. Not only are these extremely effective methods for reaching one's goals, but they also allow you to get off the boring cardio equipment in your gym and start to actually have fun while you train. Introducing these training methods will help improve your core strength, neuromuscular systems, ability to resist fatigue, and, most importantly, help you perform at a much higher level.

Greg Vandermade, MS, CSCS
Head Strength and Conditioning Coach
Cal State Fullerton

myths of all time. Sure, you DO burn a greater percentage of fat when exercising at lower intensities, but not necessarily a greater amount of total fat and calories. Using this logic, sleep might be considered the greatest fat-burning exercise of all time, right? I'll get into that in more detail in the next chapter, but there is something greater and more powerful happening with cardio strength training, and this powerful x-factor seems to be occurring AFTER the exercise is completed.

WHY DO THIS TYPE OF TRAINING?

I've already touched on this a bit, but variations of this cardio strength training or high-intensity interval-style training are extremely effective in building fitness. More importantly, it serves as an amazing fat-burning and body-transforming mode of exercise. With more and more research showing just how much more effective and efficient it is when compared to standard aerobic-style cardio, it's really becoming a no-brainer to choose this method of cardio.

WHO IS THIS TYPE OF TRAINING FOR?

The intensity of this type of exercise normally leads people to believe that it's for athletes or young people rather than the general population. This couldn't be further from the truth. I will talk about how you can manipulate interval training, even if you are a first timer or are detrained or deconditioned, and still reap the benefits of this amazing exercise protocol. Sure, it can get the competitive athlete ready for his sport's demands, but it can also help the working dad who wants to shed fat and have more energy to play with his kids.

HOW DO I PERFORM THIS TYPE OF CARDIO?

I will talk about many different methods of cardio strength training. All of them prove to be extremely effective in building fitness and shedding fat while not compromising valuable muscle mass. In Chapter 3, I will highlight all of the individual modes of cardio strength training. They can range from interval exercises using weights to calisthenics to sprints.

WHAT CAN I EXPECT?

Well, I've already touched on the all-important overload principle, so you must accept that

Cardio strength training is the foundation of our program. Our first phase of strength training is what we call functional capacity. We circuit multidirectional lunges into squat jumps into power stepups and finish with a locomotion series of skipping, leaping, jumping, and hopping. A great way to have a quantifiable measure of intensity is to check the heart rate of your athletes/clients. This number gives you a measure of how to increase or decrease the intensity of the circuits.

Todd Wright
Basketball Strength and Conditioning Coach
University of Texas

Metabolic training is not only beneficial for jacking up your metabolism, improving your VO2 max, increasing reactive strength potential, and reducing your body fat; it also has very important sport-specific applications. Pre-fatiguing an athlete with a metabolic session can be immediately followed by an anti-rotational or static core-training movement, which improves the athlete's ability to brace under duress. This allows a person to perform at a high level late in their sporting endeavor and still be able to create torso rigidity and power when needed.

Jim Smith, CSCS
Men's fitness expert
Co-Founder of The Diesel Crew
dieselcrew.com

it is not going to be easy by any means. If you have read *Men's Health Power Training*, you know just how I feel about pushing the envelope to reach your fitness goals—you need to do it and do it often. The great thing is that the human body is an amazing, resilient machine that learns to adapt and responds to overload. If you adhere to the programming and stick to the details, you can expect to see body changes you never would have believed were possible. That's a promise!

THE SCIENCE BEHIND CARDIO STRENGTH TRAINING

In the fitness community, we often hear the example of contrasting long-distance runners' physiques to those of sprinters. The long-distance runners do not do a whole lot of weight training while the sprinters tend to train quite hard in the weight room. The long-distance runners train primarily with long, steady-state aerobic activity while the sprinters stick to shorter distances or high-intensity sprint intervals. While the long-distance runners are normally far from fat, they do, for the most part, carry higher body fat percentages than the sprinters. We can't ignore genetics and body typing in this comparison, but there is something in their actual training that is causing the long-distance runners to carry more fat in spite of performing much more cardio and their greater caloric expenditure.

THE PROOF IS IN THE PROVERBIAL PUDDING

My good friend Mike Boyle, CSCS, makes a great point when he talks about various reasons why the "gym-going masses" are so out of tune with the highly effective mode of interval-style cardio. The point he makes is that from a media point of view we are inundated with elliptical machines, treadmills, and other traditional aerobic training machines and programs. People want quick fixes and an easy path to their goals. All the while the research against these methods is so glaring and one sided: from time effectiveness to fat loss to fitness improvements.

Science and research are the practitioner's best friend. They can prove that a particular type of training is ineffective, and they can also validate why certain types of training work in the real world. In the case of cardio for fat loss, the results come in loud and clear.

For example, a project conducted at East Tennessee State University in 2001 looked at two groups of obese women. One group performed steady-state aerobic work three times per week for 8 weeks, while the other group performed high-intensity interval training for the same amount of days and weeks. Both groups exercised each session until 300 calories were burned. The findings? Only the interval group improved their body composition; they also revealed no raises in resting metabolic rate in the aerobic group but increases in resting metabolic rates for more than 24 hours in the interval group. Okay, folks, let me repeat that: *The groups exercised the same exact amount in terms of caloric output, yet the interval group lost fat and raised postexercise metabolism rates while the steady-state group saw no improvements.* There seems to be something "magical" occurring in between intervals and also in the hours *after* these interval sessions.

THE #1 REASON FOR NOT EXERCISING... NOT ENOUGH TIME!

This is the number one reason people give as to why they fail to work out—not enough time. Well, here's something to ponder: Martin Gibala, PhD, a professor of kinesiology at McMaster University in Canada, found some pretty amazing results when looking at individuals performing steady-state aerobic activity versus those performing high-intensity intervals. He compared individuals performing four to six 30-second high-intensity all-out sprints on a cycle with 4-minute rest intervals to individuals performing 90 to 120 minutes of continuous moderate cycling. The researcher found no differences in exercise performance between the groups. Considering that the total training commitment for the interval group was 2.5 hours versus 10.5 hours for the continuous group, I would say that there *were* some distinct differences, wouldn't you? What makes this even more mind boggling is the fact that the interval group only actually "exercised" for 2 to 3 minutes per session

> It's now proven in the scientific realm that strength training or interval training both outperform aerobic training for conditioning and fat loss. Sadly, it's something that great coaches have known for years. What science hasn't proven yet is that a strength training–interval training hybrid outperforms both strength and interval training. Again it's something that great coaches already know. Wait for the researchers to catch up. . . .
>
> *Alwyn Cosgrove,*
> *World-renowned conditioning expert*

(versus 90 to 120 minutes per session in the continuous group), while the rest of the time was recovery. Once again, there is this "magical" occurrence I referred to earlier. Just because we have physically stopped doesn't mean our bodies are done working, thus making the argument for interval-style training for just about anyone with time constraints.

BUT I DON'T WANT TO NEGLECT MY AEROBIC FITNESS, RIGHT?

Of course you don't want to neglect your aerobic fitness. In the 2006 landmark 6-week study done by Tabata et al, comparisons in both aerobic and anaerobic capacity changes were made between continuous and intermittent high-intensity exercise groups. The now ultra-popular Tabata Protocol of 20 seconds of high-intensity work with 10-second rest intervals was compared to 60-minute sessions on spin-style bikes, and the findings shocked just about everyone in the fitness industry. The steady-state group that trained a total of 300 minutes per week showed no improvements on anaerobic capacity and a less than 10% improvement in aerobic capacity. **The interval group training less than 20 minutes per week showed a 28% improvement in anaerobic capacity and a 14% improvement in *aerobic* capacity.** Yes, you

read that correctly; the interval group had greater aerobic gains. This study proves that cardio strength training can and will improve your aerobic fitness as well!

AEROBICS FOR FAT LOSS

Probably the most significant, if not the most startling, study completed comparing steady-state training to interval training for fat loss was done by Tremblay et al in 1994. This study was similar in design to the study I referenced earlier and even goes a step further. They took two groups, having one complete 20 weeks of endurance (steady-state) training and the other complete 15 weeks of interval-style training. When all was said and done, the endurance group burned 28,661 calories via exercise while the interval group burned 13,614. That's right: The interval group burned less than half as many total calories. The researchers then adjusted for the difference in the energy cost of training and found that the interval groups lost 900 percent more subcutaneous fat than the endurance group— nine times the amount of fat.

SO IT'S A NO-BRAINER, RIGHT?

Well, you would think so, but there is such a disconnect between the gym-going public and the facts about cardio that it's still a battle to get these simple facts across. The key is that *you* are now armed with this knowledge (and you can no longer say "nobody ever told me!") and are taking the first step toward your fat-shedding, improved-fitness goals. It's still your choice; do you want to be one of the hamsters on the treadmills or do you want to be the lean, fit person in the corner getting twice the results in half the time? That's what I thought! Now keep reading; it only gets better!

CARDIO STRENGTH TRAINING MODES

The great thing about cardio strength training is the fact that it truly never gets boring! You can go for weeks and weeks without ever repeating the same cardio workout. From a psychological standpoint, this is tremendously helpful in fighting off boredom and burnout. From a physiological standpoint, this is also great as it keeps the body guessing at its ability to "adapt" and prevents the body from getting used to a particular workout session. Each session brings something new to your brain and your body; this is just one bonus to cardio strength training.

INCORPORATING WEIGHTS INTO YOUR CARDIO SESSIONS

A very effective method of cardio strength training is actually incorporating weights in either a repetition or a timed-set fashion. It is important to remember that you are after the metabolic benefits with these sessions, so the load that you choose will have to be something that you can handle for extended sets or times. I will briefly talk about the various modes of incorporating weights, as each will have its own chapter with exercises and programs.

The first mode is what I consider the "Big Daddy" of all cardio strength training methods: *complexes*. Complexes are two or more exercises performed in back-to-back fashion. For example, I may take three exercises such as a front squat, a push press, and a bent-over row. I would perform all the reps of my front squats, then move to the push press, and then to the bent-over rows to finish my set. Traditionally you would use from 5 to 10 reps of each exercise, so you can see how these can add up rather quickly to cause quite a bit of metabolic disturbance.

The next mode is called Density Training. If done correctly, Density Training is the ultimate hybrid of both metabolic and strength training. In a typical density training circuit, you would choose five exercises and load each up with approximately a 10- to 12-repetition maximum (RM). You would then perform 8 reps of each exercise in a circuit fashion for a set period of time, all the while being very conscious of your pace.

Another timed mode is what I call *on and off circuits*. These circuits are normally made up of 30 seconds of work followed by 30 seconds of rest. The loads on these sets are lighter than on the density sets since a fast pace and maximum reps are our goals in this type of scheme.

When doing intervals or circuits, remember it is always easier to do more work in short bouts than in one long workout. Interval or circuit bouts can be broken up into sets and reps in order to increase the intensity as well as the effort of the client/athlete. Intersperse stretching, core training, foam rolling, or other lower-effort drills into the high-intensity interval or circuit, and the training effect of the bout will increase as will the easy-to-overlook but critical parts of the workout that correct problems or enhance recovery.

Robb Rogers, MEd, CSCS, MSCC
Tactical Strength and Conditioning Coordinator, NSCA

Intervals are without question an exceptional method for building endurance and improving body composition. However, the biggest mistake people make is they don't choose the right intensity. To achieve the desired result from interval training, your movement must be fast and at a high intensity. Don't pace out the movement and don't choose drills that allow you to have a break within the movement. Go all out and choose exercises such as sprints, squat thrusts, rope waves, sandbag shouldering, and band upper-body drills and you too will be a believer in the power of interval training.

Josh Henkin, CS

The last type of cardio strength training that incorporates weights is Traditional Repetition sets performed in back-to-back fashion with the goal of completing all the sets in as short a time as possible. A great example of this are *24s*. 24s are a circuit of four exercises, such as squats, squat jumps, lunges, and split jumps. The goal is to push through these four exercises, each for a set of 24, and keep track of the time for completion. As you get more fit, your time will improve. I will talk more about ways to modify these, as starting with sets of 24 is normally not a good idea if you are a beginner!

"OLD SCHOOL" TRAINING

When I think of the next section of cardio strength training, all I can think of is "old school." No, not the movie, just the types of exercises you will be performing. Going back to the research done on the Tabata Protocol, we know that performing exercises in a negative rest fashion (rest periods that are shorter than the work periods) is very difficult. Due to the intensity of these exercises, I normally recommend doing them using only body weight as resistance. If I do prescribe a load, it will be something relatively light like a medicine ball or a light kettlebell that will enable you to really push the pace on your reps yet still come back to perform set after set.

Since we know that these body-weight exercises are highly effective in eliciting a metabolic response, we now need to go back to some of the old school calisthenics. These are exercises like burpees, squat jumps, clap pushups, jumping jacks, mountain climbers, etc. Yes folks, time to dust off some of these blast-from-the-past exercises. Why? Because they are some of the most butt-kicking movements ever created!

I talked about the 30–30 intervals earlier, and of course you can perform these calis-

Increasing the options available for conditioning with interval training, strength training complexes, sled training, etc., increases the likelihood that the appropriate training qualities will be focused on (speed, power, mobility, work capacity, etc.). Successful organization of this conditioning into an appropriate training plan will continue to help drive performance and fitness to new levels.

Daniel Martinez, CSCS
Strength and conditioning coach

thenics using this type of timed circuit. But since the rest is longer than the Tabata rests, it is better suited for external loads (weights). When you start getting into 20-second work and 10-second rest intervals, your body weight is generally all you can handle if you are pushing like you should be.

HEART RATE–BASED TRAINING

While I have played around quite a bit with heart rate–based interval training using a heart rate monitor, I have found that for most people it is much simpler to use timed rest periods. Heart rate–based intervals are based on your body's ability to recover. An example of a heart rate–based interval would be to perform 10 sets of 20 burpees and use your recovery heart rate to dictate when the next set would begin. We could give you a specific number based on your fitness level of, say, 110 beats per minute; you would then start your next set when your monitor showed this number. The amount of time it would take for your body to recover down to this number would vary from set to set or even day to day, for that matter. For highly trained individuals, this type of training is very effective. In the general population, I have found that timed rest periods tend to work more smoothly. One of the drawbacks of using the heart rate monitor method is that, for beginning or untrained individuals, it could take 5 minutes to get down to this heart rate level. I will talk about some heart rate–based training prescriptions later in the book for those of you who are interested in this type of training.

IT DOESN'T GET MORE BASIC THAN THIS

The last method of cardio strength training comes back to good old-fashioned Sprint Training. I know, I know—it's a kinder, gentler exercise arena these days, right? So what; it's tough to beat a good old-fashioned sprint session when it comes to creating that all-important metabolic disturbance. I will talk about all sorts of sprint interval variations, change of direction sprints, and even my chaos sport-speed drills that can be incorporated into some of the best High-Intensity Interval Training (HIIT) sessions you've tried.

The choices are almost endless and the effectiveness is unmatched. Are you ready for your journey to the best body you've ever had? As I said in the introduction, it's not going to be easy. But then again, nothing worthwhile ever is, right?

GETTING YOUR BODY READY FOR CARDIO STRENGTH TRAINING

Some of the most effective and efficient ways to ready your body for exercise involve short, simple movements. You don't need to get on a treadmill for 15 minutes to get ready for your 4-minute Tabata session.

WARMUP

The entire purpose of the warmup process is to get your core temperature high enough to cause some increase in your muscles' ability to be stretched and moved through adequate range of motion. I find that more than around 5 minutes of warm-up is overkill as the lifting complex that follows this will continue to raise the heart rate and core temperature. The mode that you choose as your warmup is up to you. Anything from a light jog on a treadmill, to jumping rope at a moderate pace, to jumping jacks, for example, will suffice. In my opinion, a 3- to 5-minute warmup of this nature works very well.

LIFTING COMPLEX

I have outlined three different lifting complexes to help you get ready for your cardio strength training sessions, a bar warmup complex, a dumbbell complex, and a body-weight complex. Two of these complexes are the same ones I used in *Men's Health Power Training*; the third is a body-weight complex for the days that you may not be in the gym for your cardio strength session. All three of these complexes are performed for 1 set of 5 repetitions per movement in a back-to-back format with no resting between movements.

An empty bar is used for the barbell complex and no more than 20-pound dumbbells are used for the dumbbell complex. Do not add external weight to the body-weight complex (i.e. wear a weighted vest, hold a medicine ball, etc.) as your body is sufficient for warmup purposes.

WARMUP COMPLEXES

BARBELL	DUMBBELL	BODY WEIGHT
Hang jump shrug	High pull	Alternating lunges
Hang power clean	Hang snatch	Squat jumps
Push press	Squat and press	Burpees
Front squat	Bent-over alternating row	Pushups
Bent-over row	Pushup	Mountain climbers
Romanian deadlift	Core row	Side squats

"GREASING THE KNEES"

A simple and highly effective method of creating more range of motion at the knees is a method often called "greasing." With this technique you simply sit into as deep a squat as possible while holding onto something stable in front of you. With your heels flat and hips down, simply move around from side to side and in a circular fashion. You will achieve more and more comfort at getting into deep squat positions the more you perform this exercise.

PERFORMING YOUR CARDIO STRENGTH AFTER A LIFTING SESSION

In this scenario, an additional warmup session will not be necessary. Your body should be ready to perform these exercises at this point, especially if you have just completed a power training–style (full-body-oriented) workout.

DYNAMIC WARMUPS

EXERCISE	REPETITIONS X DISTANCE
Knee skips	2 X 15 yards
Leg swings	2 X 10 yards
Carioca stepover	2 X 15 yards
Atlas lunge	2 X 10 yards
Lateral 180-degree squats	2 X 10 yards
Spiderman lunge	2 X 10 yards
Three-quarter-speed accelerations	2 X 20 yards

SPRINT AND AGILITY TRAINING WARMUPS

When you are getting ready to perform sprint or agility interval work, you want to make sure that you have all of your bases covered. By this I mean that you want to have your body core temperature nice and warm and have your muscles not only warmed up and loose but also ready for the explosive exercises to come. I have listed a few dynamic warmups that act as both a warmup and a flexibility tool for your high-intensity sprinting. Perform each movement for 10 to 20 yards in an up-and-back fashion (2 repetitions of each).

COOLDOWN

You will hear me state that many times you will feel like collapsing onto the floor at the end of a complex or other cardio strength-style interval; I want you to try to avoid this if you can. At the end of your session or set, you want to continue to move or, at the very least, remain standing to avoid blood pooling in your body. Your heart rate will be sky high and you will want to try to slowly lower this over the next few minutes; slow walking is the best movement for your body at this point.

At the end of your training session, a slow, light-paced jog is a great way to gradually lower your heart rate and eventually get back to a comfortable state. In fact, it may actually be an optimal time for this type of activity in terms of fat mobilization since you are coming off a tremendous metabolically-disturbing workout. An easy 5- to 10-minute jog or even a walk will do the job.

Complete 5 repetitions of each of the following movements before proceeding to the next movement. There is no rest in between movements and you will hold onto the bar the entire time.

HANG JUMP SHRUG

Holding a barbell with a pronated, shoulder-width grip, lower the weight to the top of the kneecaps by pushing the hips backward and moving the shoulders forward while keeping your back flat. (This is the "power postion.") Forcefully jump and shrug the weight as you jump off the floor. Land with feet flat and knees bent.

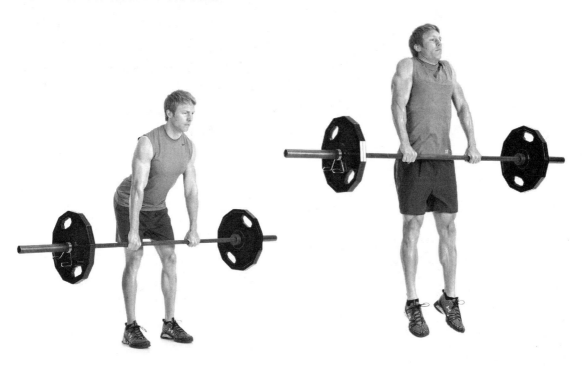

HANG POWER CLEAN

From the same position, extend and shrug the weight upward and finish by pulling the weight toward your chin. At the high point of the pull, rotate the elbows under and around the bar and catch the weight at the shoulders with the knees slightly bent.

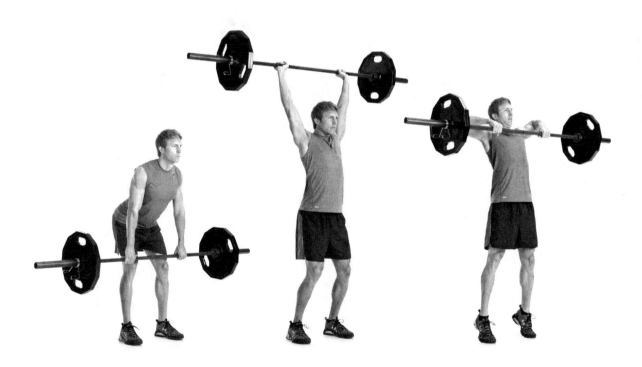

PUSH PRESS

Hold the weight at the shoulders and dip and drive the weight upward. As the bar passes your face, drop your chin so that the weight finishes overhead and above your ears. (Think of pushing the weight with the legs in this movement.)

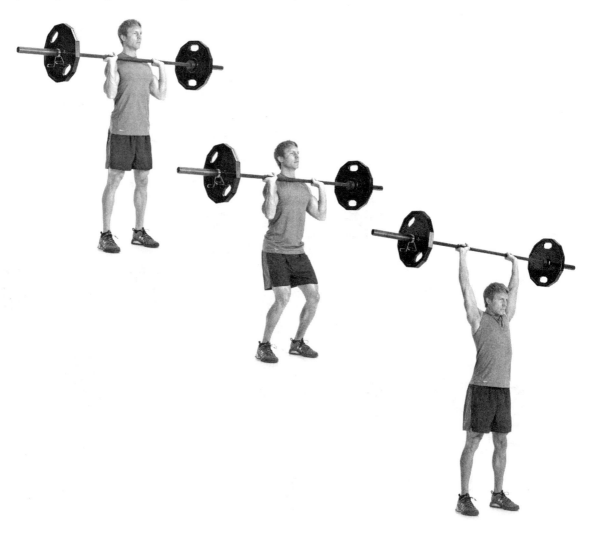

FRONT SQUAT

Sit the bar on your shoulders and open your hands up to let the bar rest firmly on your shoulders. Keeping your elbows high and your back straight, lower into as deep a squat as possible. Push the hips back so that the heels stay on the floor the entire movement.

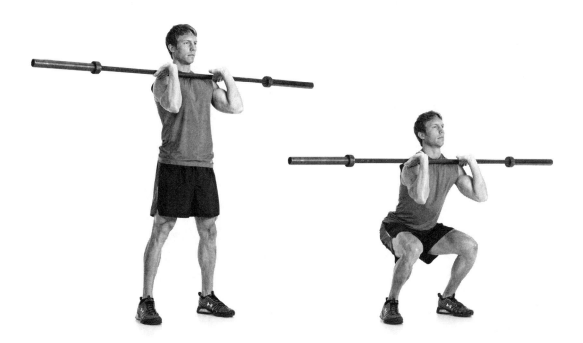

BENT-OVER ROW

Position yourself in a bent-over position by slightly bending the knees and pushing the hips back. Brace yourself with your abs and hips as you row the weight up until it touches your lower rib area.

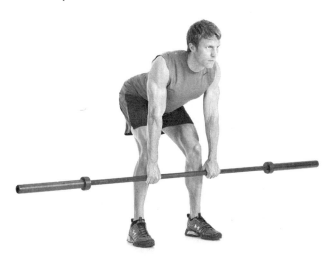

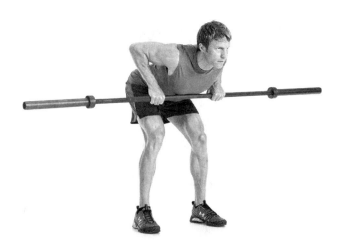

ROMANIAN DEADLIFT

Stand tall with the weight and slowly lower the bar as far as possible while keeping the knees slightly bent and pushing the hips backward as if you are trying to bump them into something behind you. Keep your eyes up and your back flat for the entire movement.

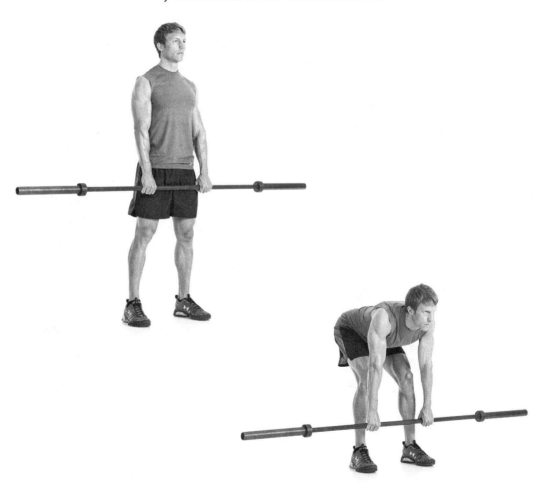

Complete 5 repetitions of each of the following movements before moving on to the next movement. There is no rest in between movements and you will hold onto the dumbbells the entire time.

HIGH PULL

Hold the dumbbells with your palms facing your legs and in "power position" as described earlier with your hips, back, and shoulders forward and knees slightly bent. Forcefully extend and shrug the weight upward, finishing with a high pull so that the elbows are high and the dumbbells end up at about shoulder height.

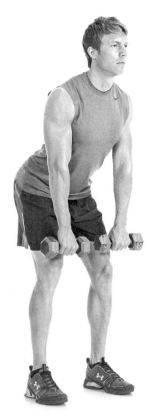
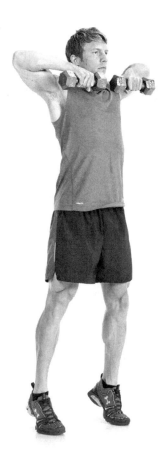

Hang Snatch

Just as in the high pull, extend and pull the dumbbells high. At the highest point of the pull, drop your hips slightly and extend the elbows so that you catch the dumbbells overhead at arm's length.

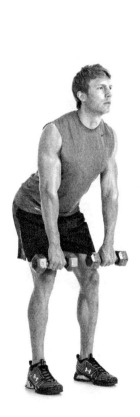
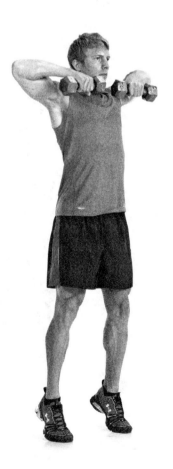
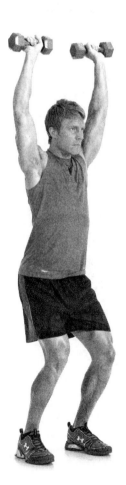

SQUAT AND PRESS

Hold the dumbbells at your shoulders with your hands in a neutral position (palms facing your head). Descend into as deep a squat as possible, then forcefully drive upward. Press the dumbbells overhead as you are coming up, using the momentum of the squat to assist in the press.

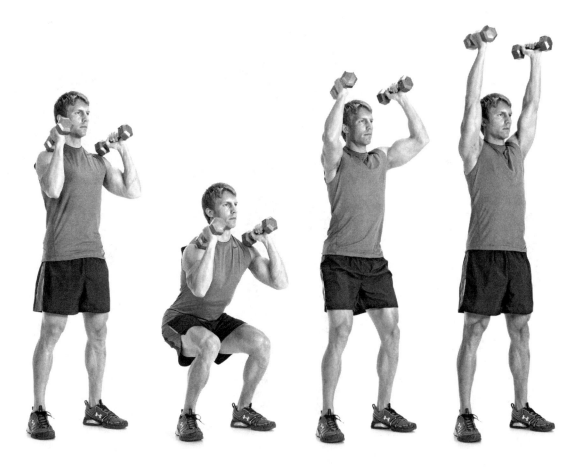

BENT-OVER ALTERNATING ROW

Set yourself in a bent-over position with back flat, hips back, and knees slightly bent. Row one arm up until the dumbbell touches your lower ribs. As you lower that dumbbell, immediately begin rowing the opposite dumbbell upward. Complete the row on both the left and right sides for 1 repetition.

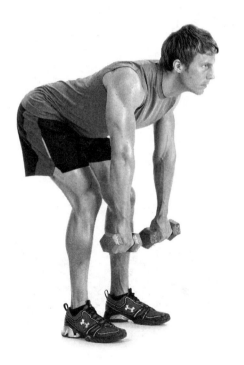 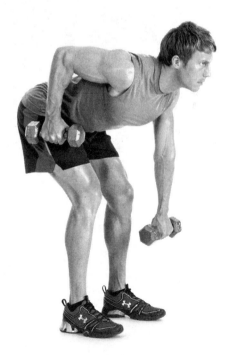

PUSHUP

Holding dumbbells in a neutral position on the floor, perform a pushup by taking advantage of the dumbbells and lower yourself farther than you would for a normal pushup.

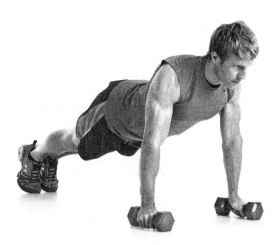

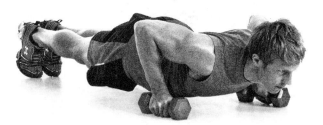

CORE ROW

At the top of the pushup position on the dumbbells, row one dumbbell up to the ribs while keeping the core tight and the body in a flat pushup position. Once the dumbbell is lowered to the floor, row the other dumbbell up. Complete both left and right sides for 1 repetition.

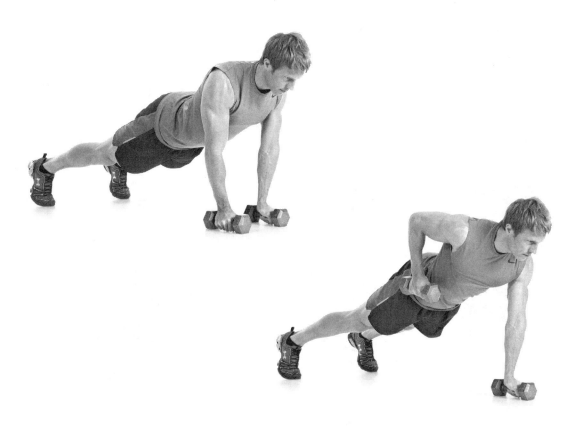

Perform 5 repetitions of each movement before moving to the next. Do not rest in between movements.

ALTERNATING LUNGES

Start with your hands at your sides and step out as far as possible while lowering the back knee until it almost touches the floor. Drive back to the start position by pushing off of your front heel before repeating on the other side. Complete both left and right sides for 1 repetition.

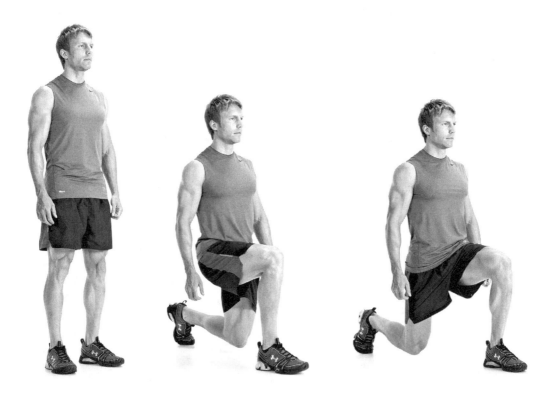

SQUAT JUMPS

Placing your hands behind your ears with your feet wider than shoulder width, squat down and explode upward as high as possible. Be sure to absorb the landing by bending the knees and immediately descending into the next squat without pausing.

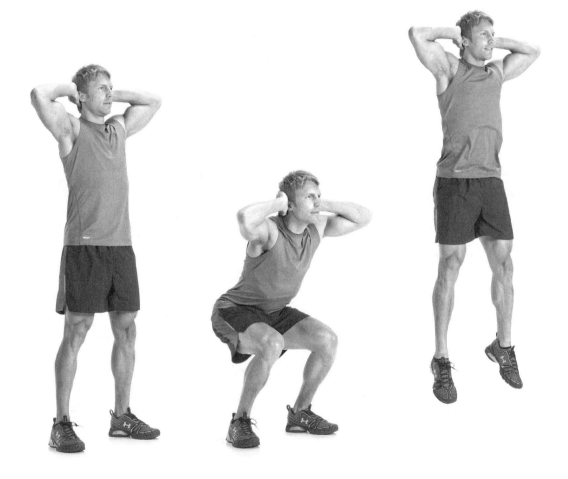

BURPEES

Start with hands at your hips, squat down to place your hands on the floor and kick out your legs until you are in a pushup position. Immediately jump your feet back underneath you and then jump out of this deep squat position back to your feet.

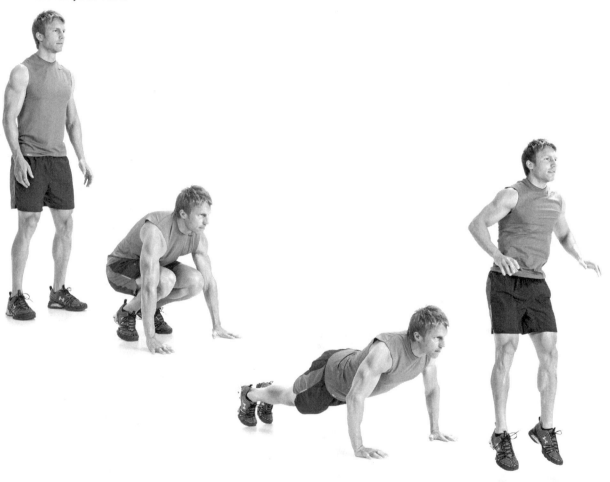

PUSHUPS

These are standard, full-range-of-motion pushups.

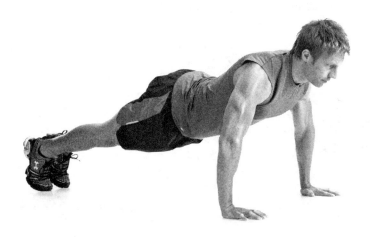

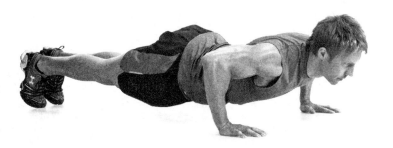

MOUNTAIN CLIMBERS

In a pushup position, take one knee and pull it into your chest so that you are balancing on your hands and one foot. Quickly switch the position of the legs by straightening the first leg and driving the opposite leg up into the chest. You should always have one foot off the ground during this exercise. Complete both left and right sides for 1 repetition.

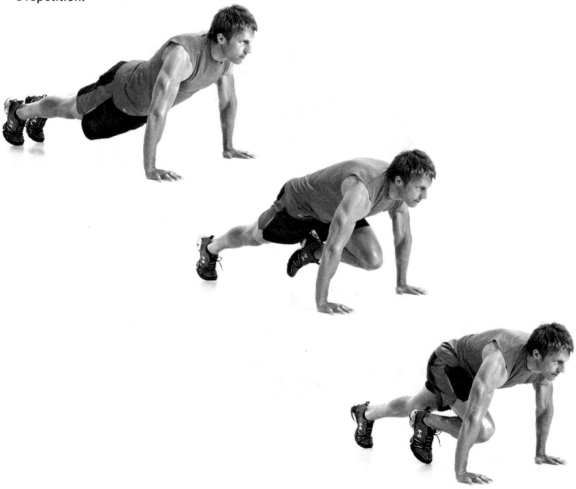

SIDE SQUATS

Stand with your feet set wide with toes slightly pointed outward and your hands in front of you. Push your hips backward as you move as far as you can to one side while keeping your feet flat on the floor. You will be in a deep knee bend position with shoulders forward and hips back as you move into your side squat. Return to the starting position and repeat on the other side. Complete both left and right sides for 1 repetition.

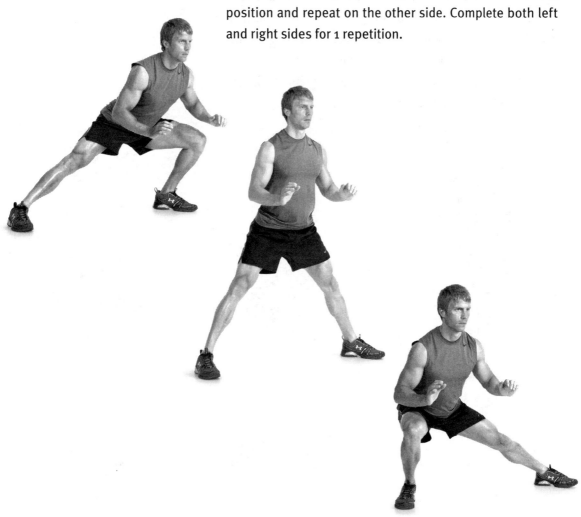

Perform each of these movements for 2 repetitions of the prescribed distance prior to your outdoor cardio strength sessions. It is important to fully warm up your body and get the muscles ready for this very taxing activity.

KNEE SKIPS (15 YARDS)

These are traditional skips where you will take off and land on the same foot before repeating on the other side. The variation here is that you should not be concerned with moving forward very fast. Rather, you want to forcefully drive the opposite knee as high as possible as quickly as possible when you skip with the other leg.

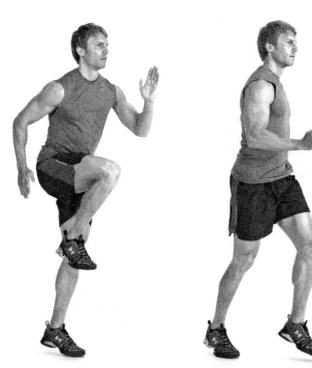
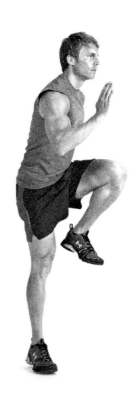

LEG SWINGS (10 YARDS)

Step and swing the opposite leg as high as possible, attempting to touch the toe with your opposite hand. Try to keep the leg straight as you swing. As the leg comes back down, let it swing backward as far as possible to help facilitate a stretch of your hip flexors as well. Keep your torso tall throughout this exercise.

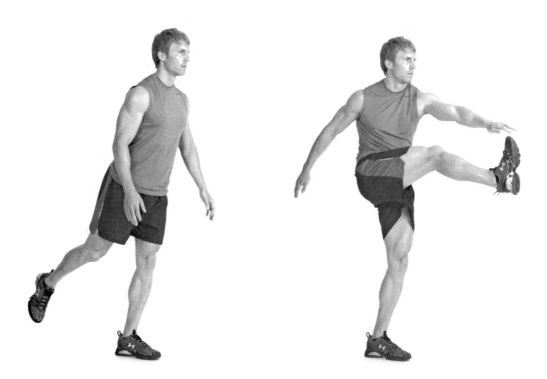

CARIOCA STEPOVER (15 YARDS)

This is a standard carioca with one variation. As you perform the crossovers both in front of and behind your body, try to pick the back knee up high as it steps around to the front of your body. It should look as if you are trying to step over your front knee.

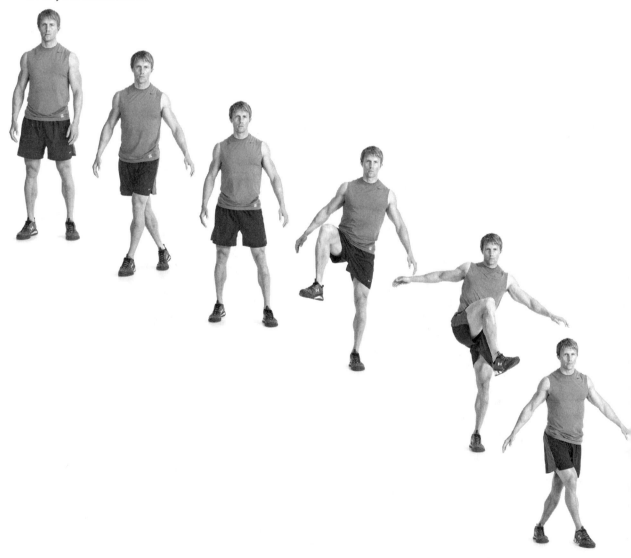

ATLAS LUNGE (10 YARDS)

Stand tall with your arms extended above your head. Step forward into a lunge and simultaneously rotate and reach backward over the same-side shoulder as you keep reaching your arms up high. You should feel a long stretch on the opposite side of your body as you descend into the lunge and rotate.

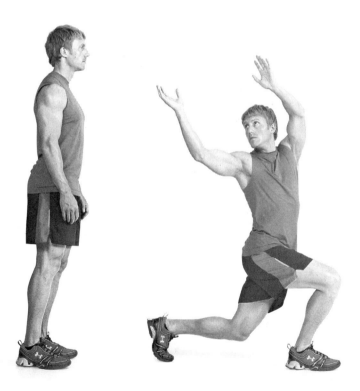

LATERAL 180-DEGREE SQUATS (10 YARDS)

Stand with feet parallel. Step out to your side as far as possible and push into a deep side squat both in that direction and back. Bring the feet back together, turn 180 degrees, and repeat in the opposite direction.

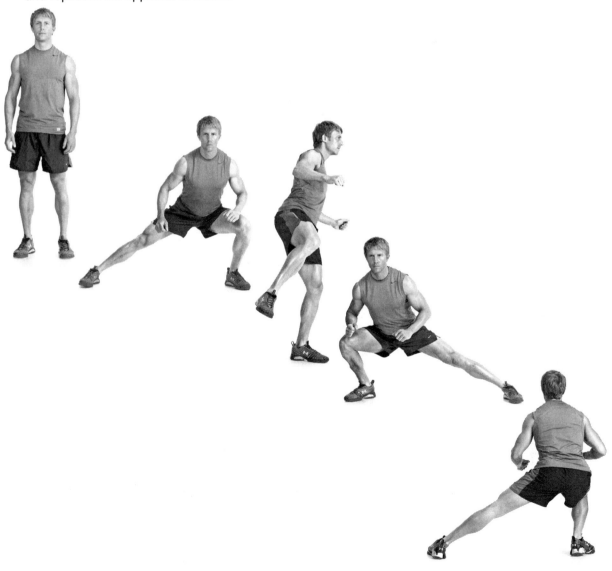

SPIDERMAN LUNGE (10 YARDS)

Starting in a bear crawl position (on all fours), step the right leg up as far as possible so that it is as close as possible to the right hand on the floor. Push into that stretch and then reach your left hand forward and attempt to step the left leg even with that hand. Keep your hips low and place the bulk of your weight on your hands to get the most out of this stretch.

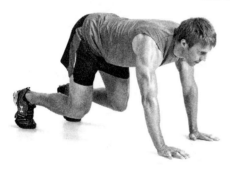

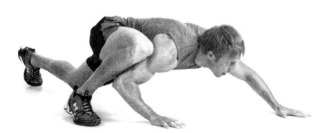

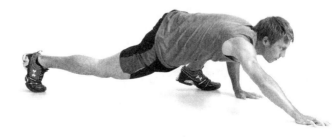

THREE-QUARTER-SPEED ACCELERATIONS (20 YARDS)

These are build-up-style runs that gradually get faster with each step you take. Start with a jog pace, then move into a stride to finish with a hard run pace. Think of trying to take large steps as you take off and run.

5

COMPLEXES

There I am, standing in front of an Olympic bar with a measly 90 pounds of load on it. I'm pacing back and forth, a million thoughts are running through my head, and my heart rate is increasing even before I do anything. Maybe I should get on the treadmill and do some hard running intervals instead of this; maybe I should do some Tabatas; or maybe I'll do my normal weight-training workout and come back to this at the end. Bottom line is that I would rather be doing just about anything other than this.

THE KING OF CARDIO STRENGTH TRAINING

What was going on in the story above, you ask? Well, I was getting ready to start my complex workout for the day. Three sets of 10 repetitions of a series of eight exercise movements all performed in a back-to-back fashion, 80 repetitions per set, 90 seconds' rest between sets. The previous scenario happens every single time I am getting ready to perform any complex workout. Even the fact that I will be actually "working" for a mere 6 minutes *total* in this session doesn't soothe my mind. The discomfort is tremendous, the anguish almost unbearable, the results unmatched. One of my favorite books is *The New Toughness Training for Sport* by Jim Loehr, EdD. In this book, Loehr talks about the concept that if there is no personal confrontation, there is no progress. Simply put, if you are not doubting yourself or not thinking of other things that you could be doing instead of the task at hand, you're probably not working hard enough on your complexes. I said it from the very beginning: Nothing worth accomplishing is going to be easy. Complexes are far from easy, but because of this they get my personal stamp of approval as the KING of all cardio strength training methods.

The Concept behind Complexes

The roots of complexes are often confusing, but the undisputed father of complexes is Istvan Javorek, a former Romanian weightlifting coach who brought these concepts over to the United States. Are complexes really that tough? Well, there is a reason one of Coach Javorek's nicknames is "Coach Javorkian"!

The setup for a complex is pretty simple. Chose two or more exercises using the same implement and load (i.e. barbell, dumbbell, kettlebell, cable, etc.), then choose your number of repetitions, sets, and load. Your exercises are then performed in a back-to-back fashion. For example, if you choose to perform a barbell front squat and a push press for 3 sets of 10 repetitions, you would perform all 10 reps of your front squats, then immediately transition to 10 repetitions of the push press. This would be 1 set. I generally like to prescribe at least three exercises in a complex, and the number of repetitions per set depends on the load that you will be using. A few simple rules need to be adhered to when performing complexes:

- Exercises should follow a smooth transition pattern.
- You cannot put down the implement until the set is completed.
- You need to determine your load based on your weakest exercise movement. By

As the father of dumbbell and barbell complexes, I am the biggest believer in these exercises. When I invented the original Javorek Complex I and Complex II in the 1970s, I was looking for something that would improve coordination, increase the workout's load, intensity, and cardiovascular quality, and in general make a program more dynamic and efficient. Over the past decades, many athletes in all sports around the world have used my complexes as a part of a complete conditioning plan.

Istvan "Steve" Javorek, undisputed creator of complexes concept
www.istvanjavorek.com

this I mean if you are going to choose something like a barbell hang snatch, overhead squat, Romanian deadlift, and bent-over row as your complex, you would most likely choose your load based on how much you can handle on your overhead squats.

You can choose to go heavy on your complexes depending on the number of exercises you choose. I personally like to stay in the 8- to 10-repetition range per set as you are really trying to tax and overload the metabolic system to cause as much metabolic disturbance as possible. In simple terms, you want to choose the number of reps that will elicit the greatest response, and then results, from your muscles. Remember that you want to push the pace so that you are unable to perform more reps at the end of your set. Choosing your loads really comes down to trial and error, once you get a feel for the movements and how long the sets take. For example, you should not have a hard time choosing the amount of weight you should use. I often tell people, "Give me a 65-pound barbell and about 5 minutes, and I guarantee I can break you."

I use a progression when prescribing complexes. We will start with fewer repetitions per set, fewer sets, and longer rest periods. Then we will progress to more sets, more repetitions, and shorter rest periods as we start to adapt and get in shape. This progression is outlined in more detail later in this chapter. Remember, this is a progressive training protocol. You cannot expect to jump into the advanced sets and complexes right away. Be patient; fitness is a journey, not a destination!

STARTER COMPLEXES

These are simple combinations that allow you to get used to choosing your loads and determining pace and rest times and so on. These are great if you have no experience with complexes and have not been exposed to interval-style metabolic training. I have prescribed three variations for each level of fitness—a barbell, a dumbbell, and a kettlebell complex. Remember that variation is a great key to your success and your psychological well-being.

Mix things up and you will be more likely to push harder and stay mentally fresh.

STARTER BARBELL	STARTER DUMBBELL	STARTER KETTLEBELL
Back squat	Front squat	Two-handed swing
Behind-the-neck push press	Push press	Sumo squat

When performing these or any of the complexes listed in this chapter, remember the rules I spoke of earlier:

- The set is not over until all of the repetitions are completed.
- The implement is never put down until the set is complete.
- Pace and load are of utmost importance— the harder you push yourself, the greater the metabolic disturbance and, in turn, the greater the fitness benefits.

BEGINNER COMPLEXES

The natural progression calls for increasing the number of exercises. Naturally, the sets will now take longer to perform since the amount of work is progressively increasing.

BEGINNER BARBELL	BEGINNER DUMBBELL	BEGINNER KETTLEBELL
Alternating lunge	Sumo deadlift	Two-handed swing
Good morning	Push press	Bottoms-Up Sumo Squat
Push press	Bent-over alternating row	Push press

INTERMEDIATE COMPLEXES

Okay, you will see that the progression is starting to result in a significant increase in workload per set. For example, using a 10-repetition set in the barbell complex listed below, even with only 65 pounds, results in a workload of more than 2,000 pounds per set. The use of a 25-pound kettlebell in the complex below results in nearly 1,800 pounds of work!

INTERMEDIATE BARBELL	INTERMEDIATE DUMBBELL	INTERMEDIATE KETTLEBELL
High pull	Curl-lunge-press hybrid	Alternating swing
Drop lunge	Romanian deadlift	Clean and press (each arm)
Good morning	Bent-over row	Windmill (each arm)
Ab rollout	Jump squat	Overhead squat (each arm)

ADVANCED COMPLEXES

This is truly the big leagues here, folks. The volumes are very high so even a very light weight will result in quite a bit of work being accomplished each and every set. Hopefully you have worked your way up to these killer complexes and now can perform them using the weekly progression shown on the opposite page.

> I find kettlebells to be exceptional for training aerobic and anaerobic energy systems concurrently. The basic lifts such as clean and jerk and snatch are full-body, multiplanar movements performed while on your feet, so in addition to working the entire neuromuscular and cardiorespiratory systems, they teach valuable athletic skills.
>
> *Steve Cotter, Director,*
> *International Kettlebells & Fitness Federation,*
> *www.ikff.com*

ADVANCED BARBELL	ADVANCED DUMBBELL	ADVANCED KETTLEBELL
Jump shrug	Hang snatch	High pull
Squat clean	Squat and press hybrid	Clean and push press hybrid
Push press		Snatch
Hang snatch	Pushup and core row hybrid	Front squat
Overhead squat	Weighted burpee	
Romanian deadlift		
Plyo pushups		

The barbell complex above is the one I was contemplating in the opening of this chapter. Using 90 pounds of load and performing a set of 10 repetitions results in over 7,000 pounds of work per set. Folks, that's over THREE TONS of work being done in around 2 minutes! If this type of work doesn't cause some of the greatest metabolic disturbance ever, I don't know what would.

COMPLEX VOLUME AND REST PERIOD PROGRESSIONS

Remember that our goal is progressive overload in just about everything we do that is fitness related. In order to accomplish this, we have to do one or more of the following things: Increase the volume (reps, sets), increase the loads, and decrease periods. Since most of the training programs are 12 weeks in duration, I have come up with a progression that increases the intensity of these complexes every 2 weeks. These sets and rest periods are not meant for the starter complexes. You should move through this progression using the beginner, intermediate, and advanced complexes as listed in the logs starting on page 211.

WEEKS	SETS X REPS	REST PERIOD
1–2	3 X 6	2 minutes
3–4	3 X 7	2 minutes
5–6	3 X 8	90 seconds
7–8	3 X 9	90 seconds
9–10	3 X 10	75 seconds
11–12	3 X 10	60 seconds

3- day lifting schedule with designated cardio strength days						
MONDAY	**TUESDAY**	**WEDNESDAY**	**THURSDAY**	**FRIDAY**	**SATURDAY**	**SUNDAY**
Lift	Cardio strength	Lift	Cardio strength	Lift	Off	Off

3-day lift without designated cardio strength days						
MONDAY	**TUESDAY**	**WEDNESDAY**	**THURSDAY**	**FRIDAY**	**SATURDAY**	**SUNDAY**
Lift complexes	Off	Lift complexes	Off	Lift complexes	Off	Off

4-day lifting schedule with designated cardio strength days						
MONDAY	**TUESDAY**	**WEDNESDAY**	**THURSDAY**	**FRIDAY**	**SATURDAY**	**SUNDAY**
Lift	Lift	Cardio strength	Lift	Lift	Cardio strength	Off

4-day lifting schedule without designated cardio strength days						
MONDAY	**TUESDAY**	**WEDNESDAY**	**THURSDAY**	**FRIDAY**	**SATURDAY**	**SUNDAY**
Lift complexes	Lift complexes	Off	Lift complexes	Lift complexes	Off	Off

RECOVERY—THE X-FACTOR

Your body's ability to recover is a direct reflection of your fitness level and, like anything, this will improve over time. The duration of your complex set completion time will have a great effect on how your body will react to the prescribed rest time. A general rule of thumb is to start with rest periods that are equal to or greater than the time it takes to complete your complex set. This is where everyone should start. Using the chart on the previous page, this means not progressing to shorter rest periods until your body adapts and can recover enough to perform the next set. In other words, it's okay to stick to 2-minute rest periods as you increase your volumes; everyone is different and we need to account for this fact.

Something that will truly tax your body is the concept of *negative rest periods*. This means that the amount of time that you rest is actually less than the amount of time it takes to complete a set. These brief rest periods are really meant for advanced trainees as they are very difficult and result in great discomfort and fatigue after each set. The ability to recover in these short periods is dependent on your fitness level, so be smart when choosing your loads and complexes when you get to the latter weeks in the above progression.

WHERE DO COMPLEXES FIT INTO MY TRAINING SCHEDULE?

Personally, I like to begin my lifting sessions with 3 sets of a complex, but many people don't like to do this as they feel worn out moving on to their weight-training workout. For these folks I recommend perhaps finishing their lifting sessions with a 3- to 4-set complex. Another option is to designate a day or two solely for cardio strength training. On these days you may do a complex, or even two different ones, and perhaps some other form of interval training.

The exact days you choose to designate as

Other tools and exercises we can use for complexing			
CABLES	BODY WEIGHT #1	BODY WEIGHT #2	SUSPENDED RINGS
Squat and row hybrid	Squats	Burpee and pullup hybrid	Horizontal rows
Woodchop (each side)	Split jumps	Squat jump	Jump squats
Split squat and press hybrid	Plyo pushups	Plyo pushups	Pushups
	Burpees	Leg raises	Ice skaters
	Mountain climbers		

cardio strength days are completely up to you. I am a firm believer in frequency as a significant factor in fitness and fat-loss benefits. Even if it's just a 15-minute interval session done one extra day per week, it is much better than doing nothing, and the metabolic disturbance that I frequently refer to will kick-start the all-important EPOC (Excess Postexercise Oxygen Consumption) factor. Strength-training expert Alwyn Cosgrove refers to this as "afterburn;" I think that's a pretty descriptive word for what is happening to your body during this postexercise period.

MORE COMPLEX TOOLS

In addition to barbells, dumbbells, and kettlebells, you can also perform complexes with body weight, medicine balls, cables, and even one of my new favorites, suspended rings. Strength coach Frank Addelia is a kettlebell, ropes, and TRX suspension system expert. Once a week we get together to "play" in what my assistant coach Dan Corbet and I like to call these sessions, the "Frank-enstein workouts." The results have been a whole new set of exercises for my cardio strength toolbox. Keep in mind that we are often limited by loads since most of these are dictated by body weight. The addition of a medicine ball, weighted vest, or even dumbbells during some of the exercises can increase the intensity. You will see many of these movements later when we talk about timed sets, but feel free to use them in complexes as they are highly effective for this method.

SOME LAST THOUGHTS ON THE KING OF CARDIO STRENGTH TRAINING

People often ask me, "What do you do during your recovery between complex sets?" My standard answer is to not say a word and to simply get down on all fours on the floor. The point is usually pretty clear when I do this. The main reason complexes are so effective is that they are THAT hard. If you are not pushing the envelope just to the brink of complete failure with each set, you are not going to get all that you can get out of these highly effective, challenging exercises.

1. BACK SQUAT

Set a barbell high on your shoulders with your feet slightly
wider than your shoulder width. Keeping your torso as
erect as possible, descend as far as you can while keeping
your heels flat on the floor.

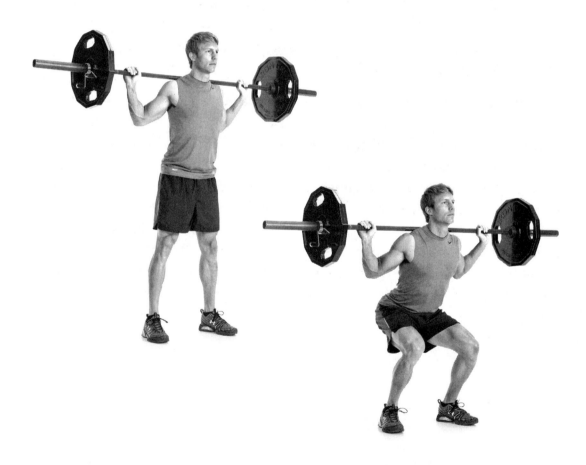

2. BEHIND-THE-NECK PUSH PRESS

With the bar high on your shoulders, dip into approximately a quarter squat and drive upward. Using the momentum from your legs, drive the weight overhead. Your arms and legs should straighten out at exactly the same time. Be sure to bend your knees as the load comes down to make contact with the back of your shoulders on the descent.

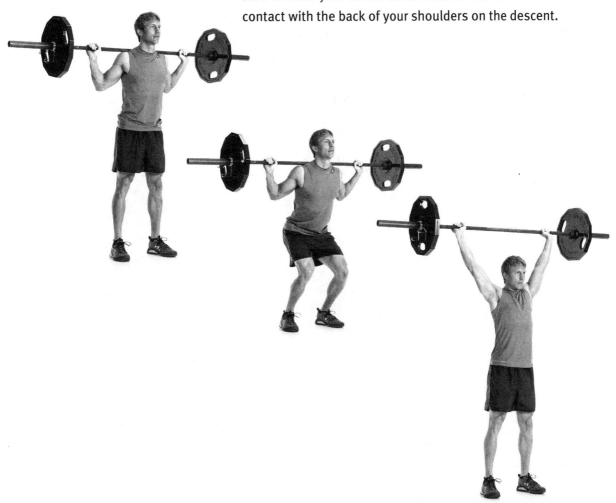

1. FRONT SQUAT

Place flat-ended dumbbells on your shoulders by setting the flat ends onto your shoulders so that your thumbs are down and palms are facing in. Your elbows should be held high and facing forward, not out to the sides. Keeping your torso as erect as possible, descend as far as you can while keeping your heels flat on the floor.

Note: *If your dumbbells do not have a flat end, you can rest the edge of the dumbbells on the front of your shoulders so that your elbows are not as high.*

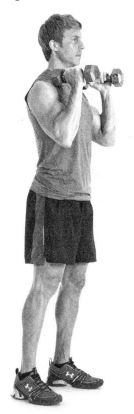
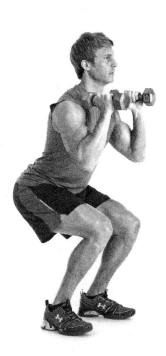

2. PUSH PRESS

With the dumbbells in the front squat position, dip into approximately a quarter squat and drive upward. Using the momentum from your legs, drive the weight overhead. Your arms and legs should straighten out at exactly the same time. Be sure to bend your knees as you lower back to the starting position.

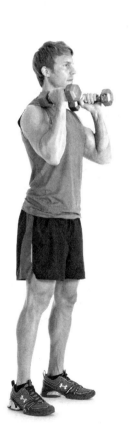
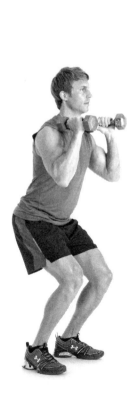
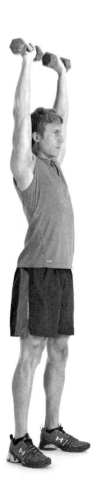

1. TWO-HANDED SWING

Holding the kettlebell with both hands and in a squat-type base, bend your knees and move your shoulders forward so that your forearms are in contact with your inner thighs. Drive the weight upward and out using the extension of your hips to move the load. Lower the kettlebell back to the starting position.

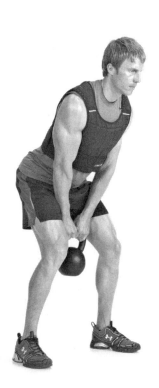
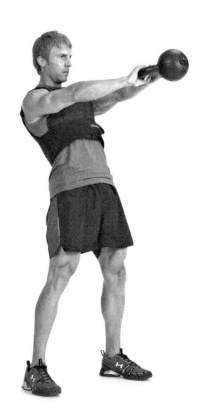

2. SUMO SQUAT

Hold a kettlebell by the handle in front of your body. Set your feet slightly wider than shoulder width with your toes pointed slightly outward. Lower as far as possible, trying to keep your torso erect and your heels flat on the floor.

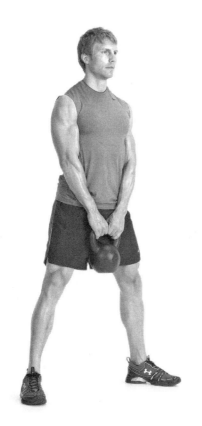
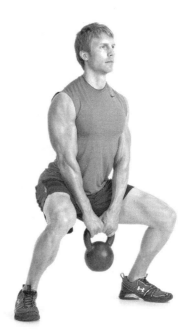

1. ALTERNATING LUNGE

With a barbell high on your shoulders and your torso erect, take a big step forward so that your heel contacts the floor first. Descend until your back knee almost touches the floor. Then drive through the heel back up to the starting position. Repeat on your other leg. One repetition is one lunge on each leg.

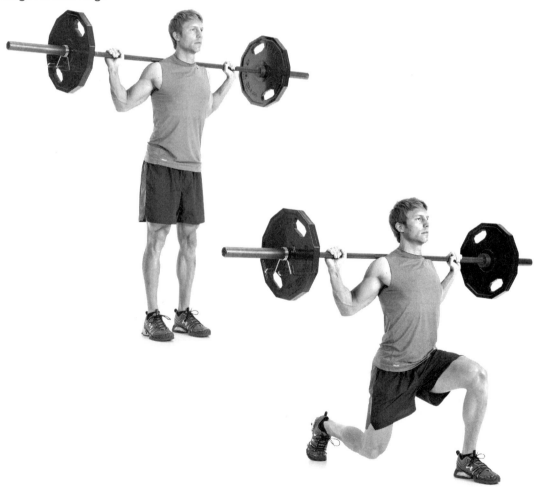

2. GOOD MORNING

With the bar high on your shoulders and feet hip-width apart, pull your shoulders back and keep your lower back slightly arched or flat. Bend your knees slightly and hold them in this position throughout the set. Begin the movement by pushing your hips back as your shoulders move forward, then descend as far as possible while keeping your eyes up and your back flat.

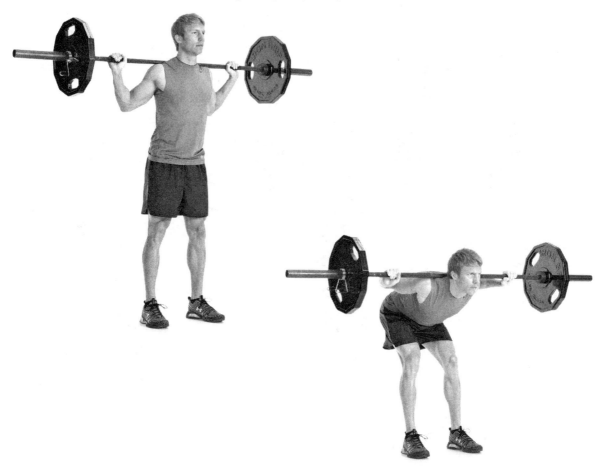

3. PUSH PRESS

With the bar high on the front of your shoulders, dip into approximately a quarter squat and drive upward. Using the momentum from your legs, drive the weight overhead. Your arms and legs should straighten out at exactly the same time. Drop your chin as the bar passes your head so that it ends up above and slightly behind your ears. Be sure to bend your knees as you lower the weight to make contact with the front of your shoulders.

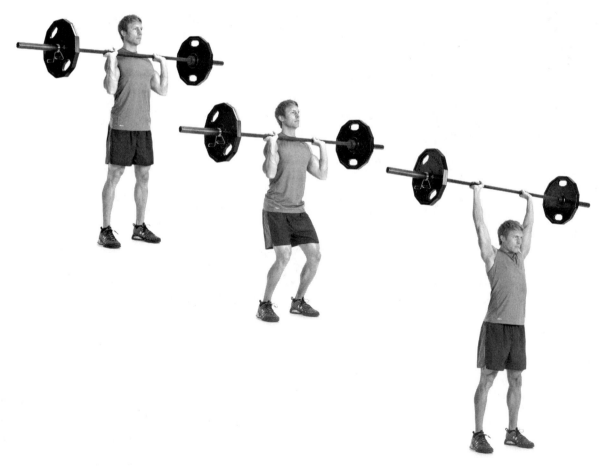

1. SUMO DEADLIFT

Hold two dumbbells in front of you and between your legs. Place your feet wider than shoulder-width apart with your toes pointed slightly outward. Lower as far as possible, trying to keep your torso erect as if you are sitting tall into a chair.

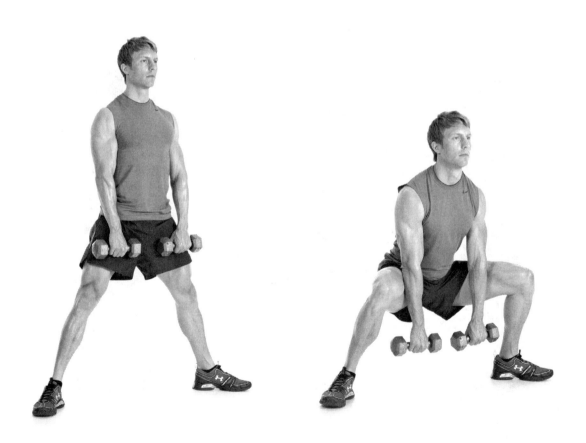

2. PUSH PRESS

With the dumbbells in the front squat position, dip into approximately a quarter squat and drive upward. Using the momentum from your legs, push the weight overhead. Your arms and legs should straighten out at exactly the same time. Be sure to bend your knees as you lower the weight.

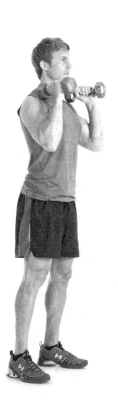
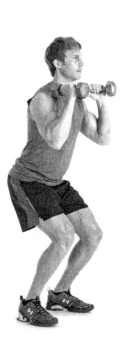
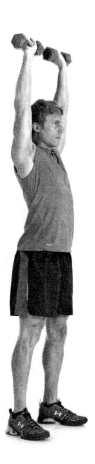

3. BENT-OVER ALTERNATING ROW

Set yourself in a bent-over position with your back flat, hips back, and knees slightly bent. Row one arm up until the dumbbell touches your lower rib cage. As you lower that dumbbell, immediately begin rowing the opposite dumbbell upward. Complete both left and right sides for 1 repetition.

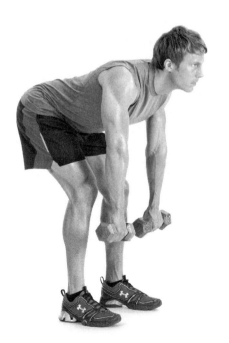
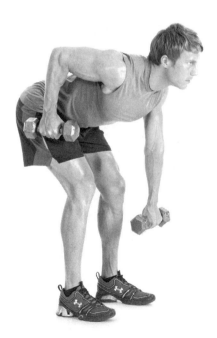

1. TWO-HANDED SWING

Holding the kettlebell with both hands and in a squat-type base as shown, bend your knees and move your shoulders forward so that your forearms are in contact with your inner thighs. Drive the weight upward and out using the extension of your hips to move the load. Lower the weight back to the starting position.

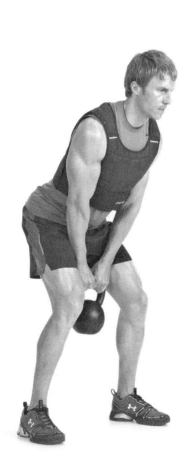
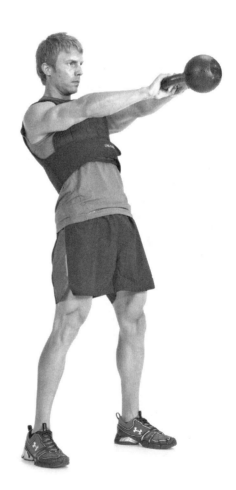

2. BOTTOMS-UP SUMO SQUAT

Holding the kettlebell upside down (heavy side up), place your feet slightly wider than hip-width apart, with your toes pointed slightly outward. Lower as far as possible, trying to keep your torso erect and your heels flat on the floor.

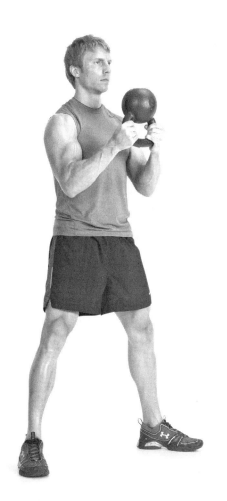

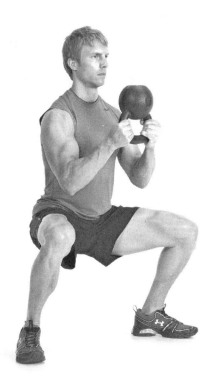

3. PUSH PRESS

Holding the kettlebells by the handle with the heavy side down this time, dip into a quarter squat and drive the kettlebells up overhead so that it ends right above your head.

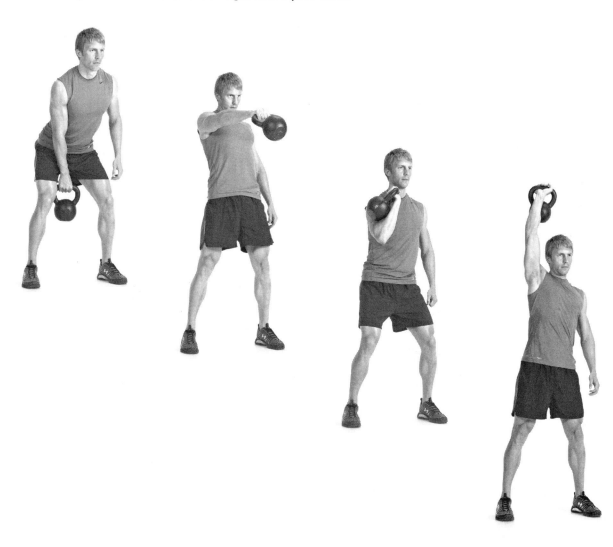

1. HIGH PULL

Starting from the floor in the pre–power clean position and with a shoulder-width grip, explode upward, keeping your back flat. As the bar passes the thighs, forcefully shrug and then continue pulling the bar with your elbows high so that you finish with the bar near your upper chest, legs extended, and up on your toes. Lower the weight carefully back down to your thighs, then lower the weight to the floor to start your next repetition.

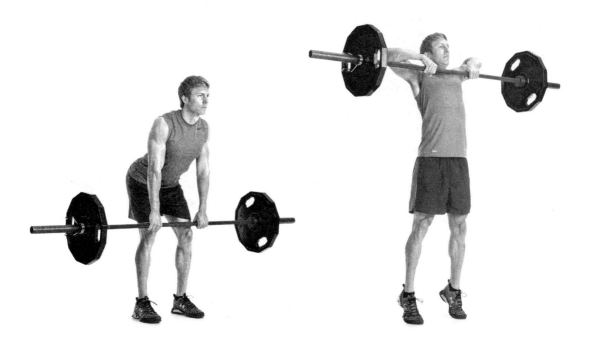

2. DROP LUNGE

Place the bar on your shoulders (behind your neck) with your feet close together. Drop one leg back and behind your body while bending your front knee to get as low as possible. Drive back up to the start position to repeat on the other side. One repetition on each side is 1 full repetition. Be sure to keep your shoulders square and your front foot pointed forward for the duration of the exercise. Let your hips do the rotating.

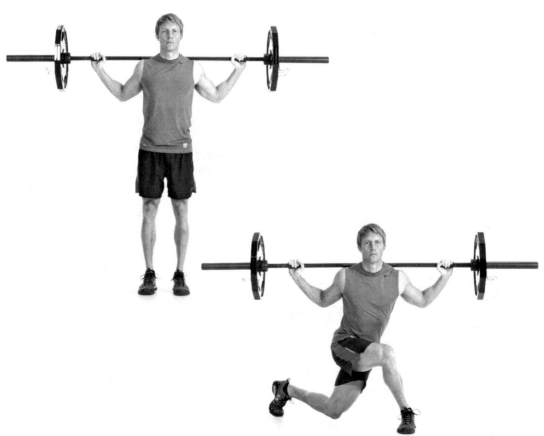

3. GOOD MORNING

With the bar high on your shoulders and feet hip-width apart, pull your shoulders back and keep your lower back slightly arched or flat. Bend your knees slightly and hold them in this position throughout the set. Begin the movement by pushing your hips back as your shoulders move forward. Descend as far as possible while keeping your eyes up and your back flat.

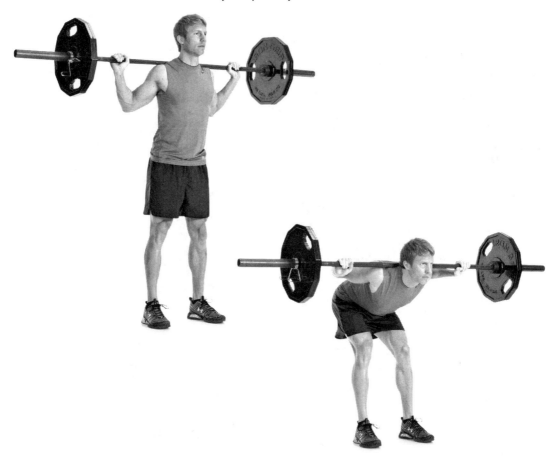

4. AB ROLLOUT

Place the bar on the floor as you sit on your knees holding the bar with a shoulder-width grip. Push the bar out by extending your arms out, then following with the hips. Roll the barbell out as far as possible before pulling back up to the start position.

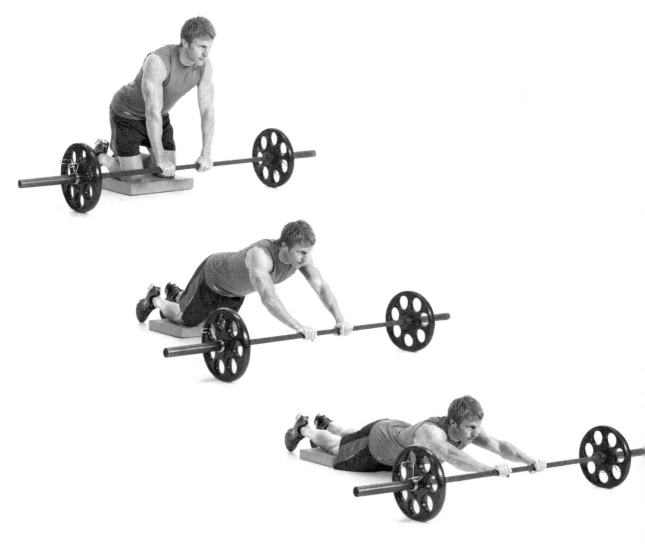

1. CURL-LUNGE-PRESS HYBRID

Hold a dumbbell at each side using a neutral grip, then step forward into a lunge. As you move forward, begin to curl the weight up to your shoulders by rotating the dumbbells so that your palms face you at the top of the curl. As your foot plants in front of you and you lower into the bottom of the lunge, simultaneously press the dumbbells overhead. Reverse the entire movement as you push back up to the starting position.

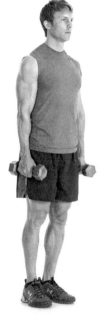

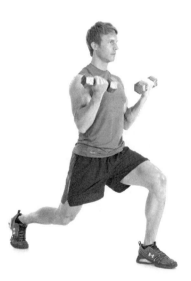

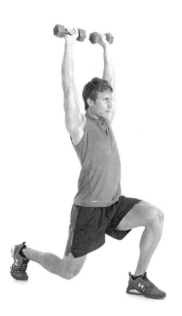

2. ROMANIAN DEADLIFT

Hold the dumbbells in front of your thighs with your palms facing your body. With your knees slightly bent, push your hips back while keeping your chest up and back flat. Lower the weight as far as possible. Think of reaching your chest forward rather than bending over to lower the weight.

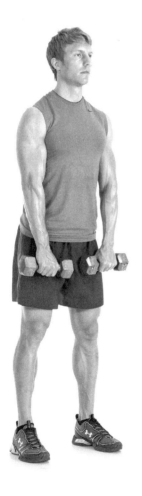
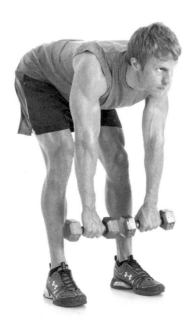

3. BENT-OVER ROW

Set yourself in a bent-over position with your back flat, hips back, and knees slightly bent. Raise the weight up until the dumbbells touch your lower rib cage.

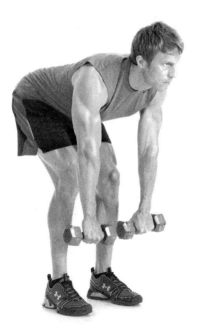
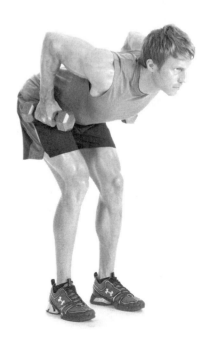

4. JUMP SQUAT

Holding the dumbbells at your sides with your palms facing your body, lower into a deep squat and explode up as high as possible, attempting to shrug the weight at the highest point. Land by absorbing the weight through your feet, ankles, knees, and hips. Then sink back into the next squat jump without pausing.

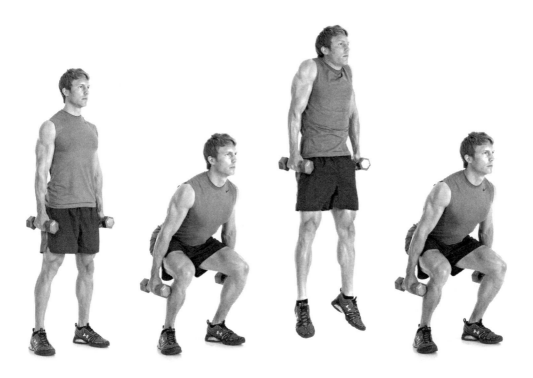

1. ALTERNATING SWING

Hold the kettlebell in one hand and lower to the power position: forward, hips back, and forearm in contact with your inner thigh. Swing the dumbbell using your hip extension to drive the weight up. At the highest point of the swing, the kettlebell will feel weightless. At this point, switch hands in midair and immediately lower the weight back to the starting position with the other arm. One repetition is a swing with both arms.

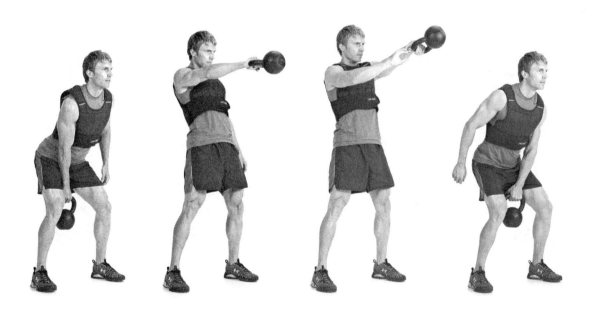

2. CLEAN AND PRESS

In the starting power position, pull the kettlebell up and quickly flip the weight over so that it is resting at your shoulder, touching both your deltoid and forearm, with your elbow down. From here, sink your shoulder and hip on that side and forcefully drive the weight overhead. Lower the weight back down to the starting position for the next rep. Complete all repetitions on one side before moving to the other side.

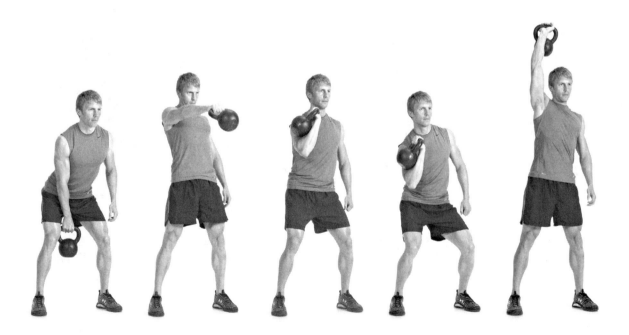

3. WINDMILL

Press the kettlebell overhead with the weight resting on the outside of your forearm. Hold your feet a little wider than shoulder-width apart with your knees almost completely locked out. Push your hips back and sideways (to the side of the kettlebell) while looking at the weight overhead and reach down to touch the floor between your feet. Perform all repetitions on that side before moving to the other side.

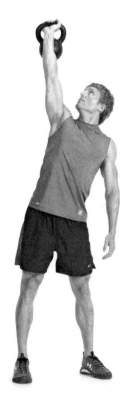
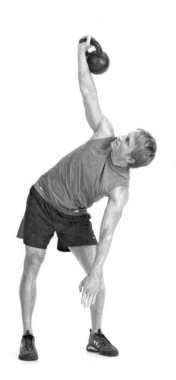
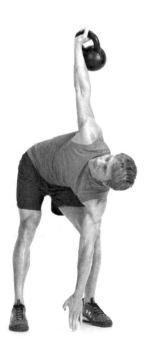

4. OVERHEAD SQUAT

Press the kettlebell overhead with the weight resting on the outside of your forearm. With your feet a little wider than hip-width apart, descend into a deep squat while looking up at the weight. Push your hips slightly toward the kettlebell side to allow a slight rotation as you squat. Keep your hips back and your heels flat on the floor throughout the entire movement. Complete all the repetions on the first side and then move to the other side.

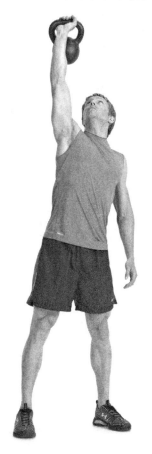
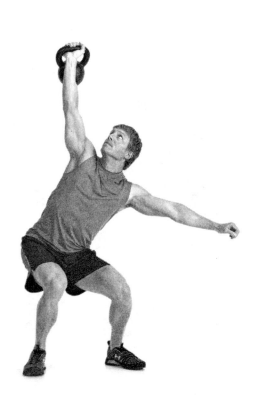

1. JUMP SHRUG

Holding the bar in the power position, forcefully jump and shrug the weight as you jump off the floor. Land with your feet flat and your knees bent.

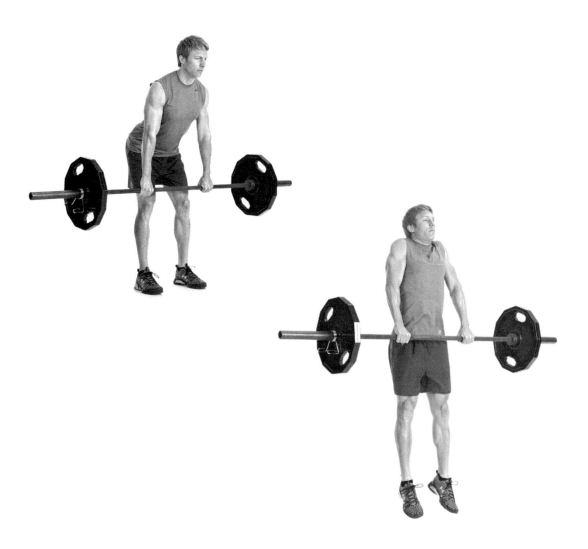

2. SQUAT CLEAN

In the same power position, extend and shrug the weight upward, finishing by pulling your arms and trying to move the weight toward your chin. At the high point of the pull, rotate the elbows under and around the bar to catch the weight at your shoulders as you drop into a deep squat position. Push the weight back up to start the next repetition.

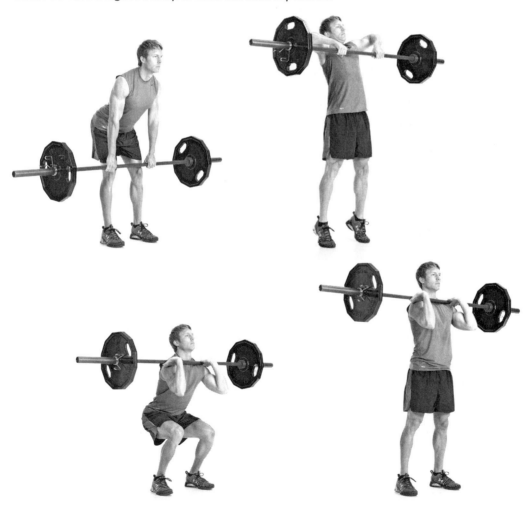

3. Push Press

Hold the weight at your shoulders, dip, and then drive the weight upward. As the bar passes your face, drop your chin so that the weight finishes overhead. Think of pushing the weight with your legs in this movement.

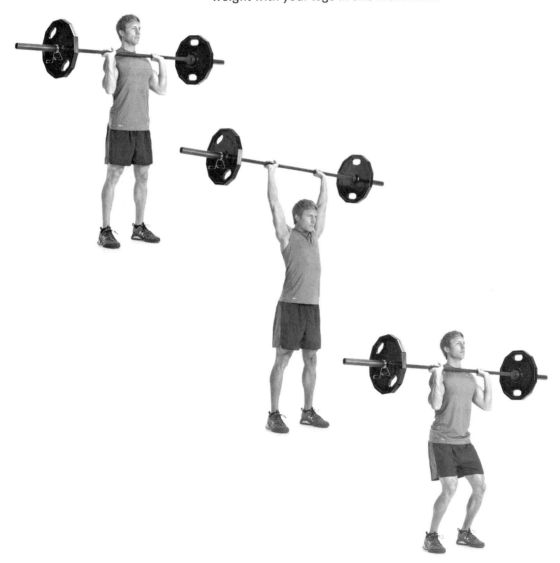

4. HANG SNATCH

In the power position using a wide grip, shrug and then jump the weight up. As the bar begins to pass your hips, continue pulling with your arms as high as possible. At the highest point of the pull, quickly extend your arms as you sink your hips down into a quarter squat. The timing should be so that your arms extend at the same time that your hips drop.

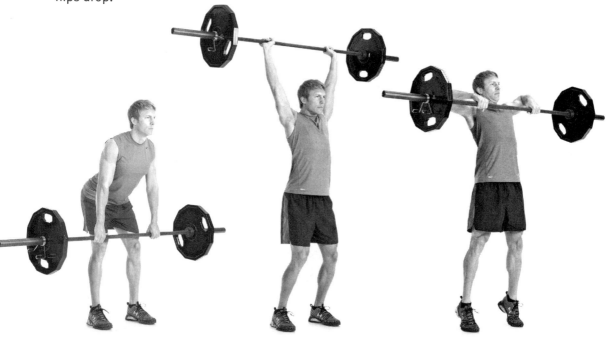

5. OVERHEAD SQUAT

With a wide grip, hold the bar above your head and slightly behind your ears. Keep your eyes and chest up as you push your hips back and descend into a deep squat while keeping your heels flat.

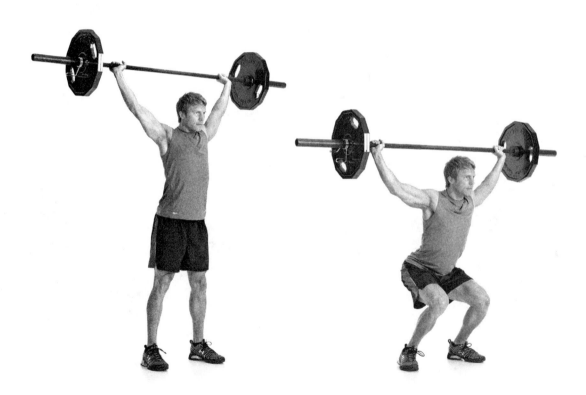

6. ROMANIAN DEADLIFT

Hold the bar with a shoulder-width grip and your palms facing your body. With your knees slightly bent, push your hips back while keeping your chest up and back flat. Lower the weight as far as possible. Think of reaching your chest forward rather than bending over to lower the weight.

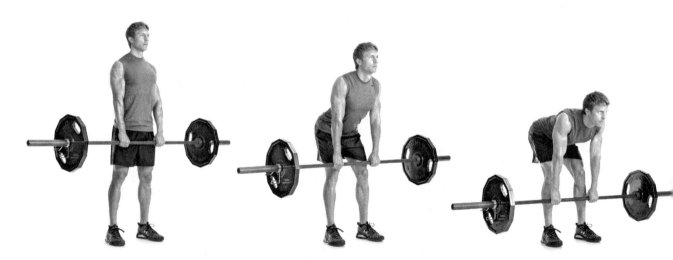

7. PLYOMETRIC PUSHUPS

Perform an explosive pushup. As your hands jump off the floor, attempt to push as far away from it as possible before landing back on the floor and moving into your next repetition. You can progress from this technique to a clap, a chest touch, an ear touch, a hip touch, and, finally, a clap behind the back.

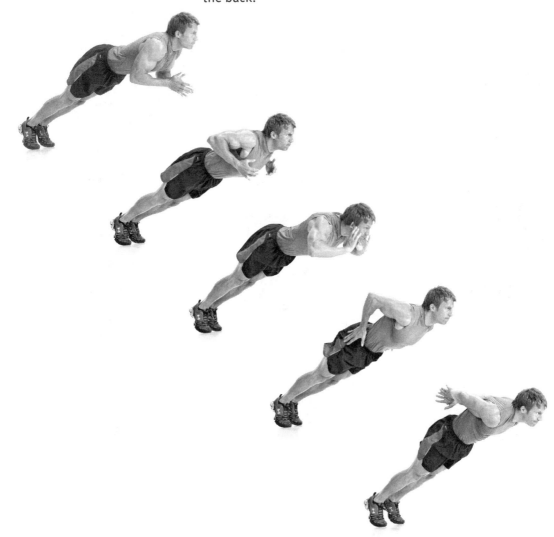

1. HANG SNATCH

Starting in the power position with your palms facing your body, shrug and jump the weight upward. As the dumbbells pass your thighs, continue pulling with your arms as high as possible. At the highest point of the pull, drop your hips slightly and extend your elbows to catch the dumbbells overhead at arm's length.

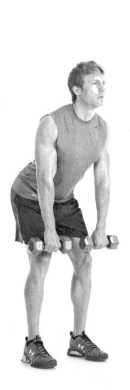
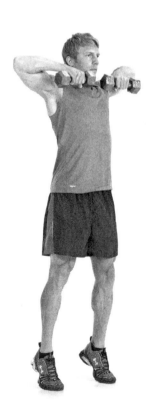
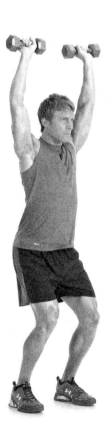

2. SQUAT AND PRESS HYBRID

Hold the dumbbells at your shoulders either with your hands in a neutral position (palms facing your head) or with the flat ends of the dumbbells resting on your shoulders with your elbows high and in front of your body. Descend into as deep a squat as possible, then forcefully drive upward. Press the dumbbells overhead as you are coming up out of the squat, using the momentum of the squat to assist you in the press.

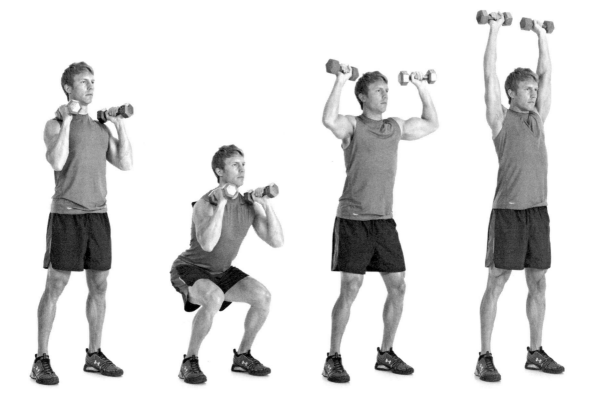

3. PUSHUP AND CORE ROW HYBRID

Place the dumbbells on the floor and perform a pushup on them. After your first pushup, row one dumbbell up to your rib cage, attempting to keep the rest of your body motionless. Lower the weight and repeat on the other side; this is 1 repetition. Avoid letting your hips rise or roll side to side.

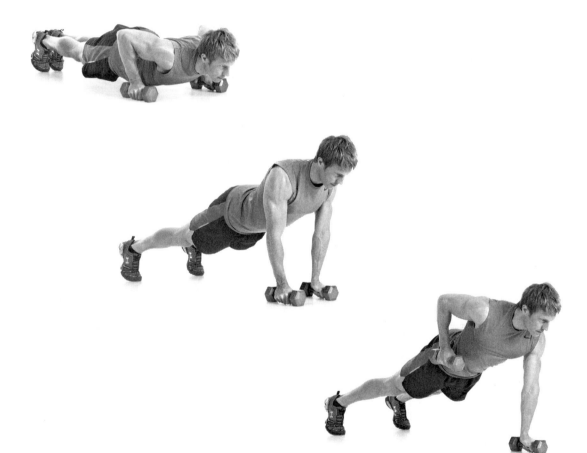

4. WEIGHTED BURPEE

Standing with the dumbbells at your sides, squat down and place the dumbbells on the floor in front of you with your palms facing in. Jump your legs out so that you are in a pushup position, then jump them back into a crouched position. Jump up as high as possible and shrug the weight at the top of the motion.

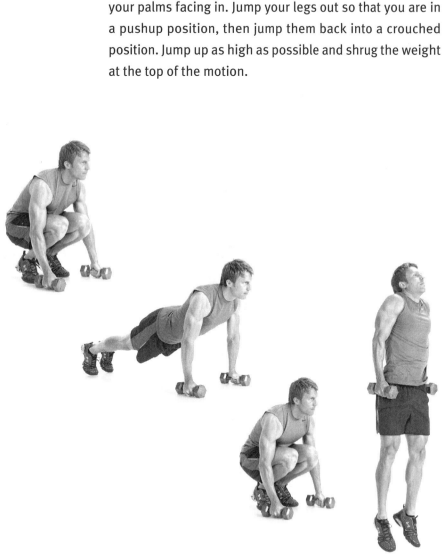

1. HIGH PULL

Hold two kettlebells in the power position. Swing the weights out and up as high as possible without letting the weight flip over your forearm. Lower the weight back down to the starting position.

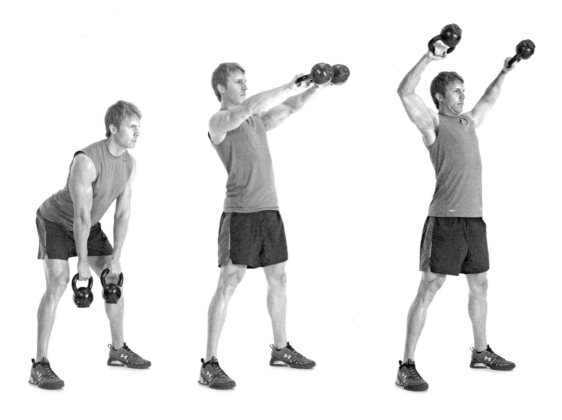

2. CLEAN AND PUSH PRESS HYBRID

In the power position, clean the kettlebells up to the shoulders and immediately dip and drive them overhead without a pause. Lower the weights back down to the power position for your next repetition.

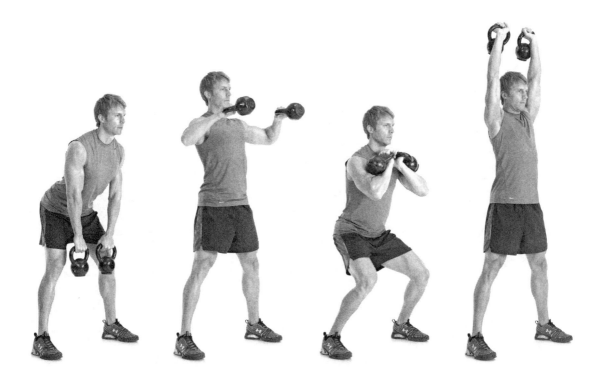

3. SNATCH

Just as in the high pull, start in the power position and swing the weight as high as possible. As the weight reaches the highest point, quickly flip it over the top of your hand and over to the other side of your forearm by flipping and punching your hand up to the ceiling. Decelerate the weight back down for your next repetition.

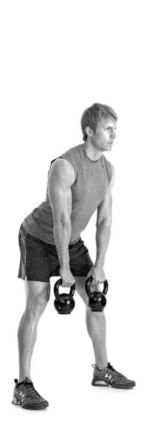 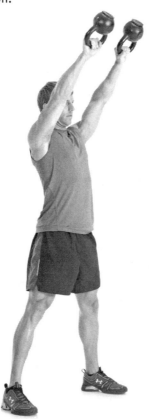 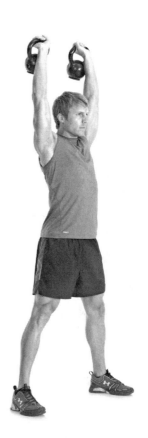

4. FRONT SQUAT

Holding the kettlebell in the clean catch position with the weight resting on both the deltoid and the forearm, descend into as deep a squat as possible, making sure to keep your core rigid and tall. Repeat on opposite side.

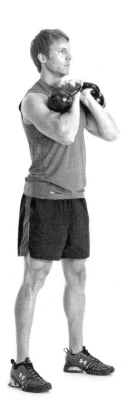
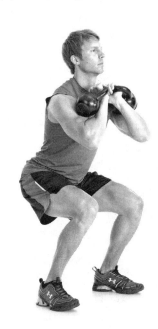

Other tools and exercises we can use for complexing			
CABLES	**BODY WEIGHT #1**	**BODY WEIGHT #2**	**SUSPENDED RINGS**
Squat and row hybrid	Squats	Burpee and pullup hybrid	Horizontal rows
Woodchop (each side)	Split jumps	Squat jump	Jump squats
Split squat and press hybrid	Plyo pushups	Plyo pushups	Pushups
	Burpees	Leg raises	Ice skaters
	Mountain climbers		

1. SQUAT AND ROW HYBRID

Holding a handle with both hands at arm's length in front of you, squat down as deep as possible while reaching forward with the arms. As you return to the start position, simultaneously row the handles back to your rib cage.

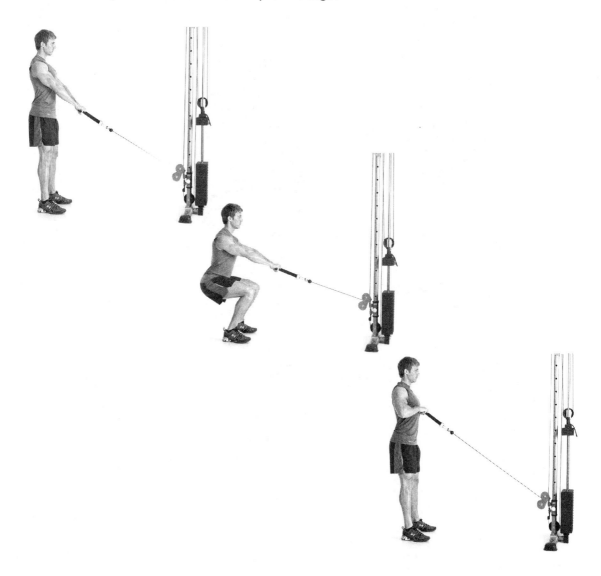

2. WOODCHOP

Hold a single handle with both hands and use either a high or a low cable position. Forcefully pull the load as you rotate your shoulders and turn your hips away from the weight stack. Be sure to pivot your back foot to facilitate as much range of motion as possible. Repeat on opposite side.

3. SPLIT SQUAT AND PRESS HYBRID

Holding the cable handle in your left hand, split your right leg forward and your left leg back. Descend into a deep split squat as you simultaneously press the handle up over-head. Perform all reps, and then turn and face the opposite direction when you switch hands.

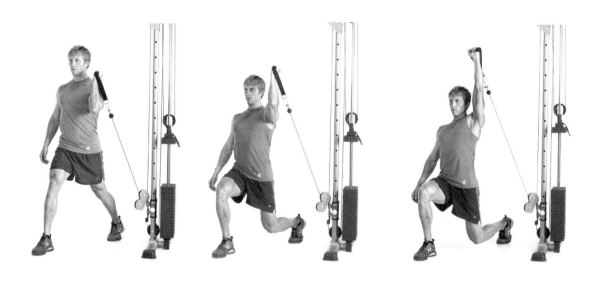

1. SQUATS

With your feet a bit wider than shoulder-width apart and
your heels flat, reach your arms forward as you descend
into a deep squat.

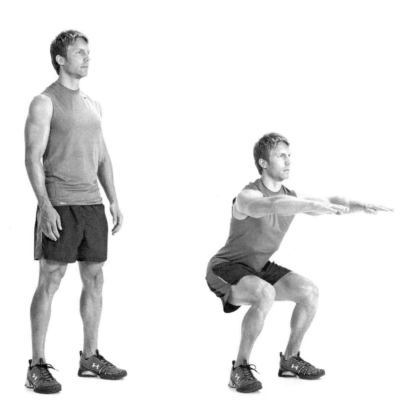

2. SPLIT JUMPS

Split one leg forward and one leg back, descend into a
deep split squat, and explode off the floor. Switch foot
positions while in the air, attempting to jump as high as
possible. Land in the opposite position and immediately
jump again upon landing.

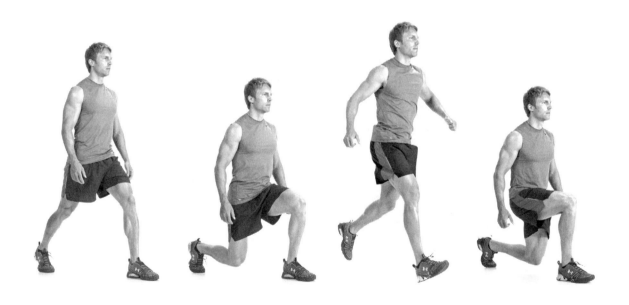

3. PLYOMETRIC PUSHUPS

Perform an explosive pushup. As your hands jump off the floor, attempt to push as far away from it as possible before landing back on the floor and moving into your next repetition. You can progress from this technique to a clap, a chest touch, an ear touch, a hip touch, and, finally, a clap behind the back.

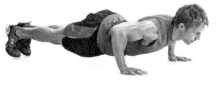

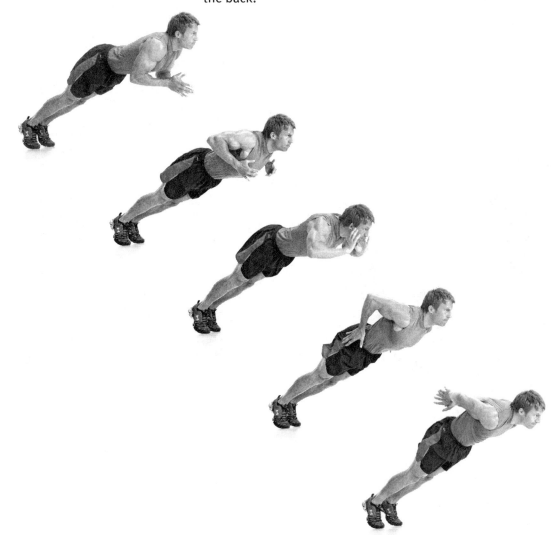

4. BURPEES

Standing tall, squat down and place your hands on the floor in front of you. Jump your legs out so that you are in a pushup position, then jump them back into a crouched position. Jump up as high as possible and reach up with your arms. Land and immediately move into the next repetition.

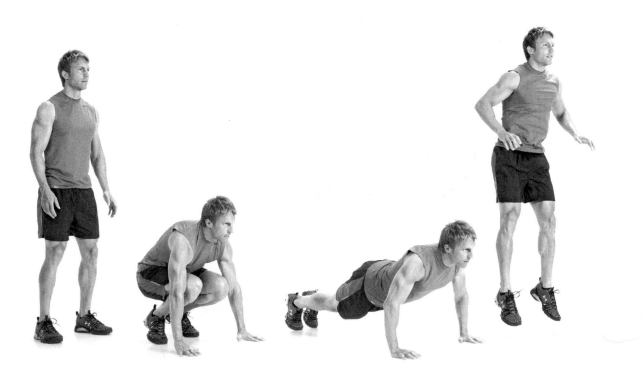

5. MOUNTAIN CLIMBERS

In a pushup position, bring one leg up so that your knee is up and pressed into your stomach. As fast as possible, switch the position of your legs, always keeping one foot off the floor. Left and right equals 1 repetition.

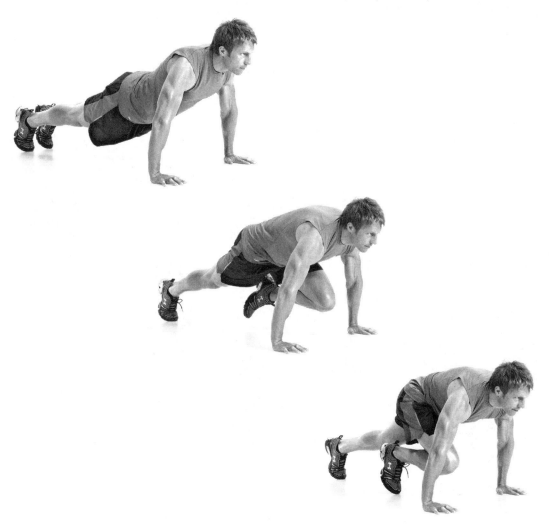

1. BURPEE AND PULLUP HYBRID

Perform a standard burpee position under a pullup bar. As you ascend out of your burpee, jump up and perform a pullup. Lower yourself under control and drop to the floor to perform the next repetition.

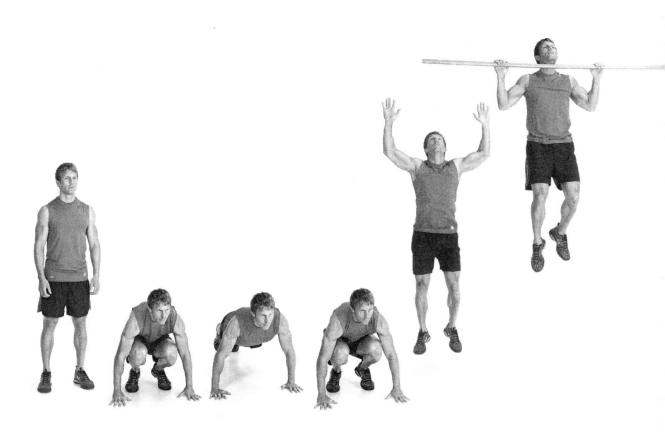

2. SQUAT JUMP

With your hands behind your head and your feet in a squatting base, descend and explode up as high as possible, making sure to absorb the impact on the landing as you sink right into your next repetition.

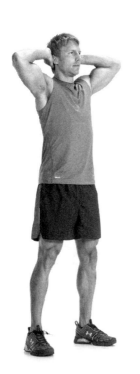
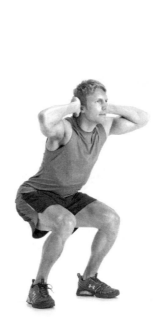
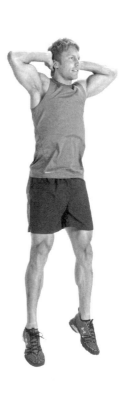

3. PLYOMETRIC PUSHUPS

Perform an explosive pushup. As your hands jump off the floor, attempt to push as far away from it as possible before landing back on the floor and moving into your next repetition. You can progress from this technique to a clap, a chest touch, an ear touch, a hip touch, and, finally, a clap behind the back.

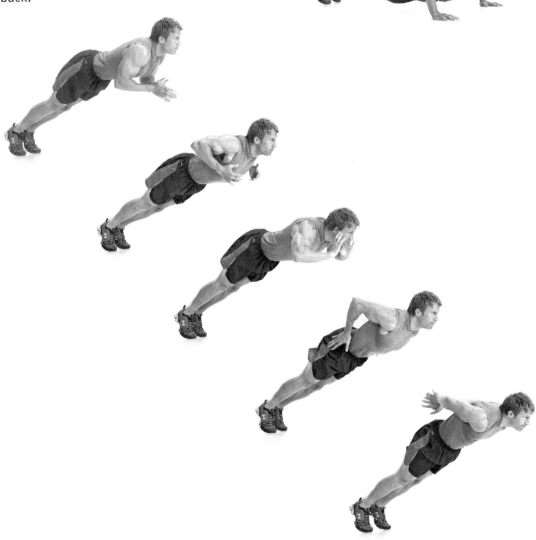

4. LEG RAISES

Using the pullup bar, swing your legs up as high as possible, attempting to touch your shins on the bar. Be sure to slightly bend your elbows and tuck your hips under to facilitate this high leg raise.

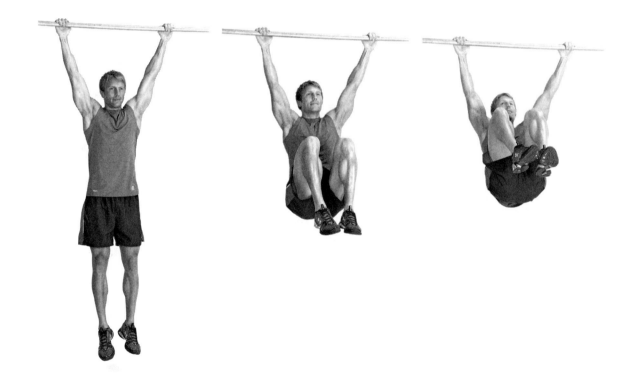

1. HORIZONTAL ROWS

Position yourself at arm's length hanging under the rings with your body rigid. How far under the rings you set up is determined by your strength. Start with your thumbs facing in and rotate your hands so that your palms are facing your body as the rings meet your rib cage.

2. JUMP SQUATS

Hold onto the rings at arm's length in front of you. Using the rings as a sort of counterweight, place your feet slightly in front of your body, sink into a deep squat, and explode upward. You will be jumping in an arcing motion. Be sure to use the rings to help you jump higher and also to help lessen the load on the descent.

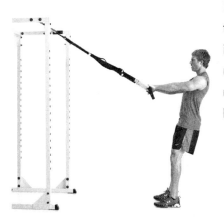

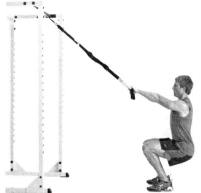

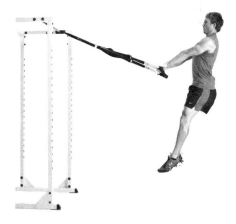

3. PUSHUPS

Hold the rings in a pushup position so that the straps are under your armpits. You can elevate your feet to make this exercise more difficult. (Placing your feet on a stability ball will make this exercise much more difficult.) Be sure to start with your palms facing your body and rotate your hands as you press up so that you end with your thumbs facing in.

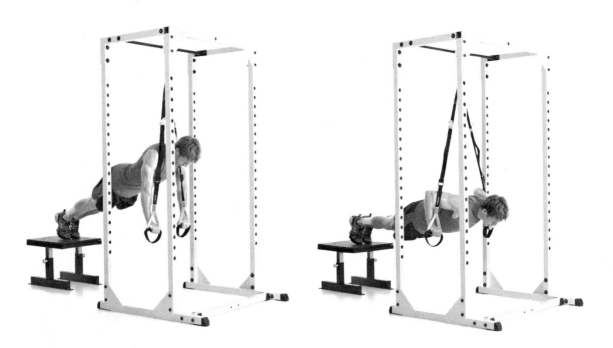

4. ICE SKATERS

Hold the rings at arm's length in front of you. Lean backward slightly as you start with your feet together. Push out to one side using your back leg to power you and reaching with the front leg. Sink into a one-legged squat as you let the trail leg sweep behind the front leg. Immediately power back in the opposite direction and repeat on the other side. Each push out counts as 1 repetition.

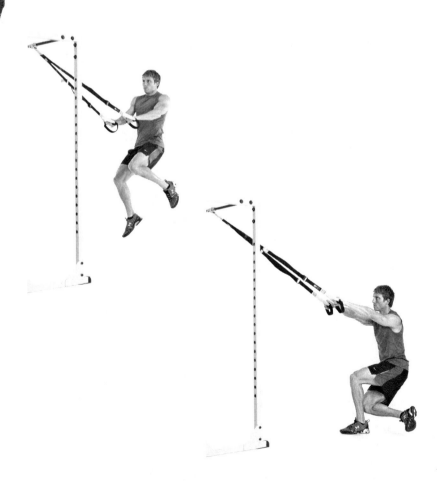

6 TIMED SETS

"Pick five exercises, load each one with your 10-repetition maximum load, perform them in a circuit fashion, and continue working for 15 minutes, trying to complete as many sets as possible." The workout seemed pretty easy when explained to me. This explanation came from Alwyn Cosgrove; the name of this type of training was called *"Density Training."* I chose dumbbell bench presses, front squats, weighted Swiss ball situps, weighted chin-ups, and dumbbell burpees as my five exercises. Fifteen minutes later I was a heaving mess of a man sitting in a corner, sweating like I just ran a marathon, and wondering what the heck had just happened and how I could be so tired so quickly. Well, I had averaged just about a set a minute, performing 8 reps per set. . . . This resulted in over 16,000 pounds of weight lifted in 15 minutes! I think we can all see now why I felt like taking a nap after this session.

DENSITY TRAINING— THE ULTIMATE STRENGTH/ METABOLIC HYBRID

Density Training is a complete hybrid of both metabolic training and strength training. Unlike in complexes, the goal in Density Training is more strength based yet the outcome, from a metabolic standpoint, is still quite similar. If I had the time to do only one method of training, I would definitely choose density sessions as my main exercise mode. The loads that we are using are in the strength and hypertrophy training ranges, yet the pace of our training builds work capacity and fitness very quickly. Let's take a closer look at Density Training.

CIRCUIT SETUP

First off, I want to acknowledge where much of my Density Training concept came from. My friend Charles Staley created something he called EDT, or Escalating Density Training, where the amount of work you do is pushed to the limit based on time constraints. This type of training is very easy to quantify, which makes even the smallest bit of progress easy to identify.

The way I set up my density sessions involves the following rules:

- Choose five exercises, one from each of the menu lists.
- Pick a weight that is your approximate 10- to 12-repetition maximum for each exercise.

- Move from exercise to exercise in a circuit format.
- Move as fast as you can through the circuit, resting as much as you need to along the way. Your goal is to get as close to averaging a set per minute as you can.

If you are moving at a much faster pace than this, the loads you have chosen are too light; if you are not even close to this pace, the loads are too heavy. As you play around with the different exercises and loads, you will start to develop a sense of the optimal loads to choose for each exercise.

DENSITY TRAINING EXERCISE MENU

EXPLOSIVE	KNEE DOMINANT	UPPER BODY PUSH	UPPER BODY PULL	CORE
Jump squat	Front squat	Split squat	Pullups	One-arm dumbbell plank row
Seated pause box jump	Back squat	Bench press	Chinups	Spiderman pushups
Kettlebell alternating swing	Overhead squat	Incline press	Side-to-side pullups	Standing barbell anti-rotation
Kettlebell snatch	Bulgarian split squat	Dumbbell alternating bench	Horizontal pullups	Barbell situps
Jump shrug	Drop lunge	Dumbbell half bench	Suspended rows	Cable woodchop (low to high)
Hang clean	Single-leg squat	Push press	One-arm horizontal pullup	Cable woodchop (high to low)
Hang snatch		Push jerk	Bent-over row	Cable push-pull anti-rotation
Dumbbell burpees		Dumbbell push press	Cable face pulls	Ab rollout
Bulgarian split jump		Dips		Windmills
		Suspension pushups		

DENSITY EXERCISE MENU

The density menu has five categories: Explosive, Knee Dominant, Upper Body Push, Upper Body Pull, and Core. The knee-dominant, upper-body-push, and upper-body-pull exercises are fairly clear cut when it comes to how much weight you're using. With the explosive exercise, you really want to choose something that is taxing to complete for 8 reps, but not taxing to the point where your form or ability to generate substantial power is compromised. The core exercise works best with something that requires an appropriate load and can be done with repetitions; in other words, things like bridges and other planks aren't as good for this circuit.

You will choose an exercise from each menu category, then decide on the amount of weight you want to use. Start the clock using either a 10-, 15-, or 20-minute session to see how many sets you can complete in this time period. Pick an order and stay in that order for the entire time period. When

"Preestablished time limits put your motivation into warp-drive; knowing that you'll be done in 20 minutes, you'll be willing to work harder than you would with an open time frame. Also, by controlling the variable of duration, you'll get a better handle on whether or not you're truly making progress.

Charles Staley, author and creator of Escalating Density Training (EDT)

you get very fatigued, rest as much as you need to, but remember that your goal is to complete a set per minute on average. Also remember that if you choose a unilateral exercise like lunges, for example, this will take longer to complete since you have to perform all the reps on each leg per set. Keep track of your sets or rounds (a round is a completion of the entire five-exercise sequence) and alter your loads based on how many sets you were able to complete on subsequent density workouts.

EXPLOSIVE	KNEE/HIP DOMINANT	UPPER BODY PUSH	UPPER BODY PULL	CORE
Seated pause box jump with dumbells*	Single-leg squat*	Dumbbell incline	Chinups with vest*	Ab rollout with band*
Dumbbell burpee	Overhead squat	Push press	One-arm dumbbell core row	Cable woodchop (high to low)
Jump shrug	Drop lunge	Dumbbell half bench	Cable face pull	Weighted ball situp
Bulgarian split jump	Dumbell one-leg Romanian deadlift	Dips with weight vest*	Side-to-side pullup	Barbell situp

Note: These exercises take longer to complete.

For those of you who perform several Density Training sessions per week, I suggest alternating between choosing a knee-dominant and a hip-dominant exercise each session. I have listed a menu of hip-dominant exercises below.

HIP DOMINANT
Romanian deadlift
Good morning
One-leg back extension
Dumbbell one-leg RDL
Seated good morning
Stability ball leg curl
Val slide leg curl

Keep in mind that the highlighted exercises on page 111 will take longer to complete, as you will have to complete all the repetitions on each limb or switch sides to complete the repetitions on the other side. As I mentioned earlier, try to limit the amount of these types of exercises during density sessions. My recommendation is to never include more than two of these in one session for the purpose of time.

COACH DOS'S FAVORITE DENSITY EXERCISE COMBINATIONS

Here are four of my favorite combinations for density sessions. You will notice that I add

difficulty by supplementing with weighted vests, dumbbells, and mini-bands on certain exercises.*

TIMED SETS WITH LONGER REST INTERVALS

Another cardio strength training variation using timed sets involves having a work interval with a longer rest interval to allow for greater work to be accomplished during work period. A very simple work-to-rest interval that I like to use is a 30-second to 60-second protocol. This creates a 90-second work bout (remember from the studies that our bodies are still working during these longer rest periods). As we get in better shape we will progress to longer work intervals and shorter rest periods. What I like to do is create a circuit of exercises and move through them in order, similar to the density circuits. Here is an example of one of these longer rest interval circuits. You would perform each exercise for 30 seconds straight then rest for 60 seconds before moving to the next exercise movement. You would decide how many rounds you are to complete based on your fitness level etc.

TIMED SET USING 30 SECONDS WORK: 60-SECOND REST INTERVAL	
SAMPLE CIRCUIT #1—BEGINNER	**SAMPLE CIRCUIT #2—ADVANCED**
1. Reverse lunge	1. Split squat (pause 3 seconds at bottom)
2. Pushup	2. Other leg forward
3. Plank walkup	3. Pushup (pause 3 seconds at bottom)
4. Split squat jump	4. Plank with weight transfer
	5. Squat jump (pause 3 seconds at bottom)

THE 30/30 TIMED INTERVALS

Another favorite of mine when it comes to timed sets is a simple yet extremely effective 30-second work/30-second rest interval. You can do this using 10-, 15-, or 20-minute time periods. Just remember that however many minutes you choose to go will result in that same amount of sets of work being completed (i.e., 15 minutes equals 15 work sets of 30 seconds). These are similar to the density sets, but the objective in these intervals is more pace than it is load. With the density sets, you rest as long as needed at times so that you can complete the next set successfully. With the 30/30 intervals, loads are lighter and your objective is to add more repetitions per set as you get in better shape. I have highlighted a sample sequence for a kettleball, barbell, and body weight circuit for this 30/30 interval.

COACH DOS'S FAVORITE 30/30 INTERVAL EXERCISE LIST		
KETTLEBELL	**BARBELL**	**BODY WEIGHT**
Alternating swings	Jump shrug	Burpees
Snatch (each arm)	Push press	Alternating lunges
Windmill (each side)	Good morning	Pushups
Front squat (each side)	Bent-over row	Mountain climbers
Push press (each arm)	Front squats	Squat jumps
Sumo jump squat		
10 minutes = one time through	10 minutes = two times through	10 minutes = two times through
20 minutes = two times through	20 minutes = four times through	20 minutes = four times through

Remember that you need to be selective with your loads so that you are able to work continuously for the entire 30-second interval.

THE 40:20 TIMED INTERVALS

The toughest progression in these timed interval protocols is the 40 seconds of work: 20 seconds of work protocol. This negative rest protocol calls for work intervals that are longer than the rest intervals. This is a great way to start to improve your recovery and work capacity to an even greater extent than the 30:30 intervals. It is important to understand that since the work intervals are longer with shorter rest intervals that your pace or tempo will have to slow a little bit in order to complete the workout. You want to be far removed from your comfort zones but at the same time you want to be able to work continuosly throughout the 40-second work interval. I have outlined some of my favorite 40:20 interval exercise combinations below.

TIMED SETS WITH 40 SECONDS WORK: 20 SECONDS REST		
SAMPLE #1	SAMPLE #2	SAMPLE #3
Val slide atomic pushup	TRX atomic pushup	Medicine ball split lunge jump
Kettlebell swing	TRX wakeboard jump	Medicine ball pushup
Val slide ab slide	TRX rows	Medicine ball straight leg situp
Kettlebell alternate swing	TRX one-leg squat jumps	Medicine ball overhead squat
Val slide sled push	TRX ab reach	Medicine ball burpees

As a bonus, I have created, along with BJ Gaddour, CSCS, and Topher Pharrel, CSCS, some custom 30/30 tracks. Visit coach dosmusic.com to download your free track.

TIMED SETS WITH LONGER REST INTERVALS

Another cardio strength training variation using timed sets involves having a work interval with a longer rest interval to allow for greater work to be accomplished during the work period. A very simple work-to-rest interval that I like to use is a 30-second to

TIMED SET USING 30-SECOND WORK TO 90-SECOND REST INTERVALS	
SAMPLE CIRCUIT #1—BEGINNER	**SAMPLE CIRCUIT #2—ADVANCED**
1. Reverse lunge	1. Split squat (pause 3 seconds at bottom)
2. Pushup	2. Other leg forward
3. Plank walkup	3. Pushup (pause 3 seconds at bottom)
4. Split squat jump	4. Plank with weight transfer
	5. Squat jump (pause 3 seconds at bottom)

90-second protocol. This creates a 2-minute work bout (remember from the studies that our bodies are still working during these longer rest periods). As we get in better shape, we will progress to longer work intervals and shorter rest periods. What I like to do is create a circuit of exercises and move through them in order, similar to the density circuits. Below is an example of one of these longer rest interval circuits. You would perform each exercise for 30 seconds straight, then rest for 90 seconds before moving to the next exercise movement. You would decide how many rounds you are to complete based on your fitness level.

ONE LAST TAKE ON THE TIMED SET CONCEPT

You can just as easily perform similar circuits as the ones listed above using a set number of repetitions rather than a set amount of time. The most popular example is the infamous "24s"; 24s are a sequence of exercises each done for 24 repetitions with the goal being to improve your time to completion. Below is the exercise sequence for 24s; keep in mind that you want to perform good repetitions (full range of motion, good form, etc.) for all repetitions before moving on to the next exercise. Since we are targeting very specific muscle groups here, the fatigue will be extreme. A simple progression would be to start with 10s, then 12s, then 15s, and so forth, until you are able to complete all the 24s without stopping.

24s
Squats
Squat jumps
Lunges (each leg)
Split squat jumps

One of my all-time favorite repetition counting circuits are what I call "countdowns." Countdowns are a combination of squat jumps and plyometric pushups done in a descending order. For example, you would perform 10 plyometric pushups, immediately move to your feet and perform 10 squat jumps, then rest for a 10-second count. You would then do this sequence with 9 repetitions of each and so on until you finish with 1 repetition of each. To make things more difficult in this exercise, eliminate the 10-second rest after you reach 5 repetitions—yikes!

You can just as easily take either of the circuits listed in the "longer rest interval" chart on page 113 (or any circuit of exercises) and pick a set number of repetitions to complete. Simply keep track of your time for completion, and now you have a fairly sound tool to check your fitness progress as well.

WHERE DO TIMED SETS FIT INTO MY REGULAR LIFTING SCHEDULE?

I like to take a density or a 30/30 interval session and make that the entire focus for one session. A 20-minute session of either of these will pretty much wear you out, and starting a session already fatigued will result in a poor workout. Try to either replace a regular lifting day with a 30/30 interval session or simply do them on days that you don't have a regular lift scheduled.

Something short like a set of 24s or "countdowns" can easily be done at the end of any training session as what I like to call a "finisher." Think of finishers as one more log on your metabolic fire just for good measure.

COUNTDOWNS	PLYO PUSHUPS	SQUAT JUMPS	REST
Set #1	10	10	10 seconds
Set #2	9	9	10 seconds
Set #3	8	8	10 seconds
Set #4	7	7	10 seconds
Set #5	6	6	10 seconds
Set #6	5	5	No rest
Set #7	4	4	No rest
Set #8	3	3	No rest
Set #9	2	2	No rest
Set #10	1	1	Done!

20/10S

Choose two lower body exercises and two upper body exercises. You will perform 20 reps of the lower body exercises and 10 reps of the upper body exercises in an alternating fashion for up to five times total.

Here's an example:

20 Burpees/Squat thrusts
10 Pushups
20 Squat jumps
10 Inverted rows
Repeat five times

If performed five times, you'll do 100 burpees, 100 squat jumps, 50 pushups, and 50 inverted rows.

This will be guaranteed to get your heart rate up and cause a metabolic disturbance. If you're an advanced athlete, you can choose exercises with loads (weight vest, dumbbells, barbells, kettlebells, sandbags, and so forth).

Brijesh Patel, CSCS
Head strength and conditioning coach,
Quinnipiac University

INTRODUCTION TO THE WORLD-FAMOUS TABATA PROTOCOL

From the introduction and the research chapter, you are now pretty familiar with the Tabata Protocol. I want to briefly touch on this protocol since it does fit into the concept of timed intervals. The biggest difference between these Tabatas and the density sessions (and even the 30/30 intervals) that I have described in this chapter is the rest intervals. Tabatas rely on negative rest intervals; these are rest periods that are actually shorter than the work intervals. Needless to say, this results in extremely difficult interval repetitions as the session progresses. Because of this, I personally prefer to use little to no external load when performing Tabatas. In the next chapter I will talk about my favorite exercise sequences for Tabatas and different progressions, but in this chapter I want to give three examples of using external loads (kettlebell, barbell, and dumbbell) in a Tabata protocol. Remember that you will perform eight rounds of 20 seconds of all-out work followed by 10 seconds of rest for a total of 4 minutes.

KETTLEBELL	BARBELL	DUMBBELL
Two-handed swing	Front squat + Push press	Sumo squat + Curl and press

Choose a weight that you will be able to continuously lift throughout the entire work interval. Perform this exercise as fast as you can, shooting for at least 12 to 15 repetitions

I love the AirDyne bike for my Tabata interval training. If you are talking "maximum metabolic disturbance with minimal muscular disruption" as the great Alwyn Cosgrove says, then AirDyne Tabatas are the best.

Try this protocol:

Six rounds using the 20/10 Tabata (2:50)
Rest 3 minutes
Repeat with another six rounds using the 20/10 Tabata

Try to get over level 10 every time and try to get 1 mile each time. It will be the hardest thing you ever did.

Mike Boyle, world-renowned strength and conditioning specialist

per interval. These are extremely difficult work intervals and this is why I will give you lots of great body-weight Tabata sequences in the next chapter.

JUMP SQUAT

Place the bar behind your head on your shoulders. Lower into a deep squat and explode up as high as possible, attempting to pull the bar down onto your shoulders so that it doesn't bounce as you jump. Attempt to land by absorbing the impact through your feet, ankles, knees, and hips, then sink back into the next jump squat without pausing.

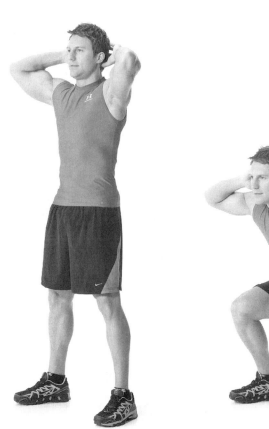
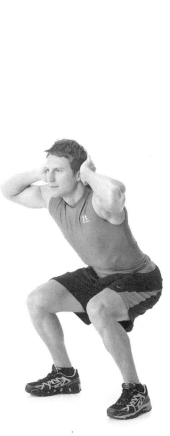
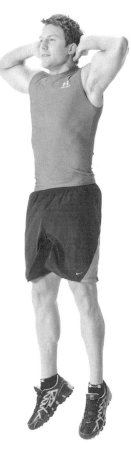

SEATED PAUSE BOX JUMP

Sit on a bench facing a sturdy box and place your hands behind your head or across your shoulders. After sitting for a few seconds, jump up as fast as possible without rolling forward and land on top of the box. Step down and sit back on the bench to get ready for your next rep. You can make this exercise more difficult by lowering your sitting position using a smaller bench/step or even sitting on a medicine ball. In addition, you can hold weights on your shoulders or wear a weighted vest.

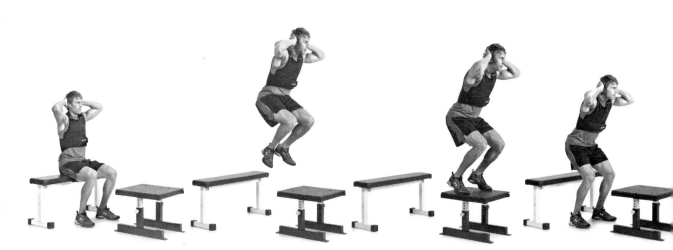

KETTLEBELL ALTERNATING SWING

Hold the kettlebell in one hand and lower to the power position with your shoulders forward, hips back, and forearm in contact with your inner thigh. Swing the dumbbell using your hip extension to drive the weight up. At the highest point of the swing the weight will feel weightless; at this point switch hands in midair and immediately decelerate the weight back to the starting position with the other arm. One repetition is a swing with both arms.

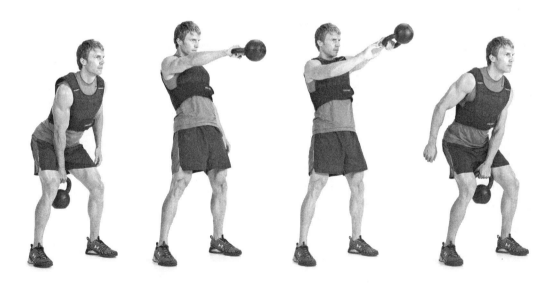

KETTLEBELL SNATCH

Using one or two kettlebells, start in the power position
and swing the weight as high as possible. As the weight
reaches the highest point, quickly flip the weight over the
top of the hand and over to the other side of the forearm by
flipping and punching your hand up to the ceiling. Decelerate the weight back down for your next repetition.

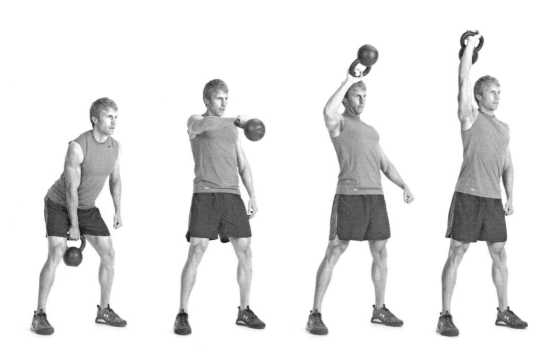

JUMP SHRUG

Holding the bar in the power position, forcefully jump and shrug the weight as you jump off the floor. Land with your feet flat and your knees bent.

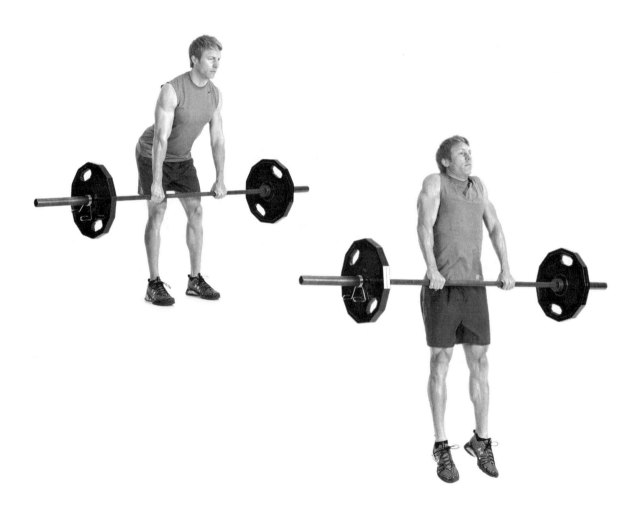

HANG CLEAN

In the power hang position, extend and shrug the weight upward while finishing with a pulling of your arms, trying to move the weight toward your chin. At the high point of the pull, rotate your elbows under and around the bar and catch the weight at your shoulders as you drop into short quarter-squat position.

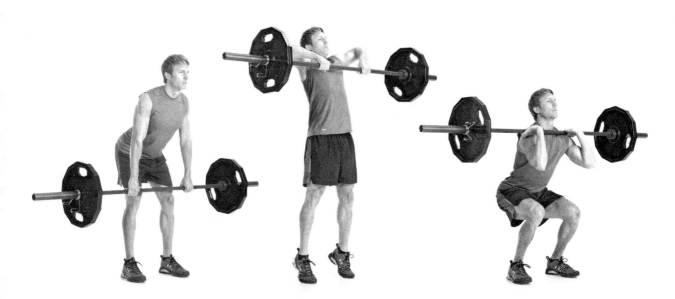

HANG SNATCH

In the power position using either a wide grip or a clean grip, shrug and jump the weight up. As the bar begins to pass the hips, continue pulling with your arms as high as possible. At the highest point of the pull, quickly extend your arms as you sink your hips down into a quarter squat. The timing should be so that your arms extend at the same time your hips drop.

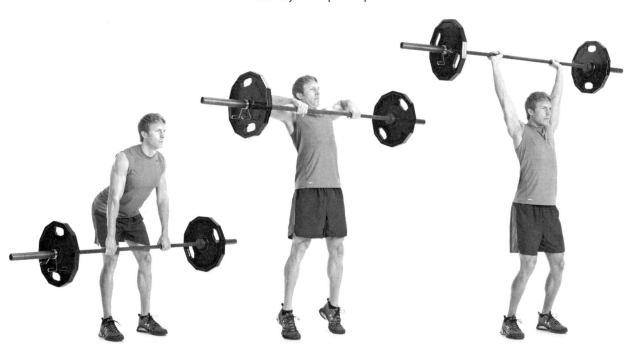

DUMBBELL BURPEES

Standing and holding the dumbbells at your sides, squat
down and place the dumbbells on the floor in front of you
with palms facing in. Jump your legs back so that you are in
a pushup position, then jump them forward into a crouched
position. Jump up as high as possible, attempting to shrug
the weight at the top of the motion.

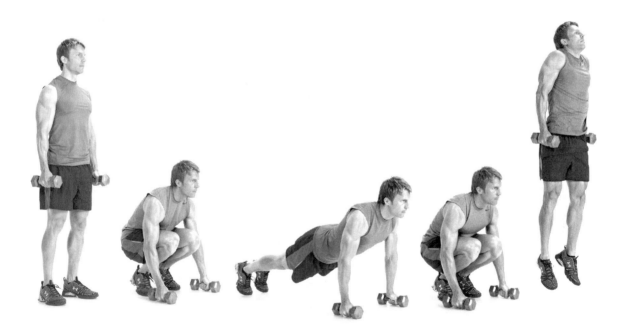

BULGARIAN SPLIT JUMP

Stand with one leg split out in front and the other foot elevated on a bench behind you. Be sure to place the front leg far out in front of your body. Descend into a deep Bulgarian split squat and then explode up, attempting to raise your front knee as high as possible in front of you. Absorb down into a deep squat before performing the next repetition without hesitation. Repeat the repetitions on the other leg.

FRONT SQUAT

Using a clean grip, cross grip, or straps, keep your elbows high as you descend into a deep squat. Try to maintain similar back and shin angles throughout the lift, keeping your heels flat on the floor.

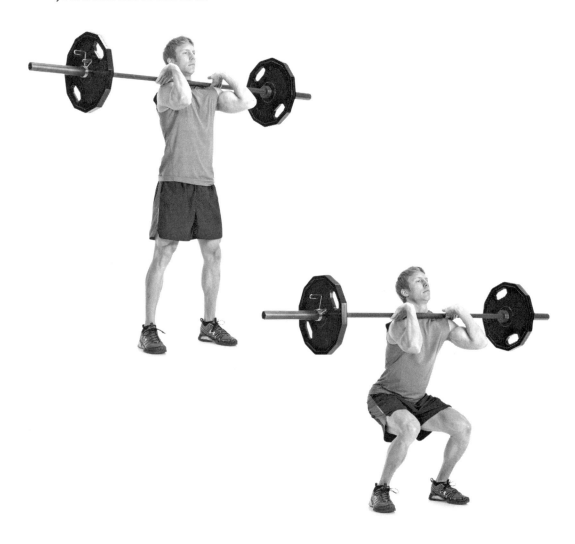

BACK SQUAT

Set the bar high on your shoulders with your feet slightly wider than shoulder-width apart. Keeping your torso as erect as possible, descend as far as you can while keeping your heels flat on the floor.

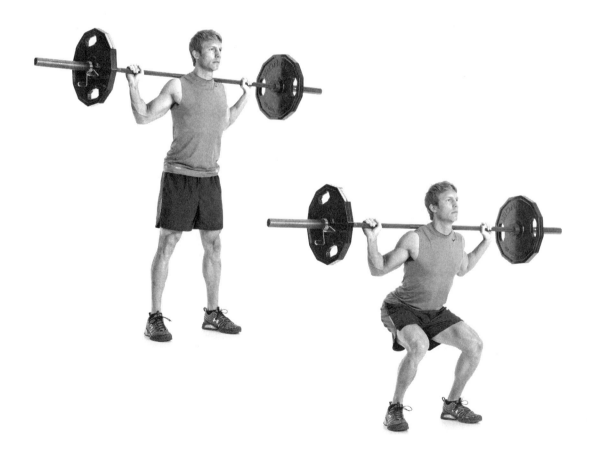

OVERHEAD SQUAT

Use a wide snatch-style grip, holding the bar overhead and slightly behind your ears. Keep your eyes and chest up as you push your hips back and descend into a deep squat. It is normal for the torso to lean forward during these squats, but try to keep your core tight and your heels flat through-out the lift.

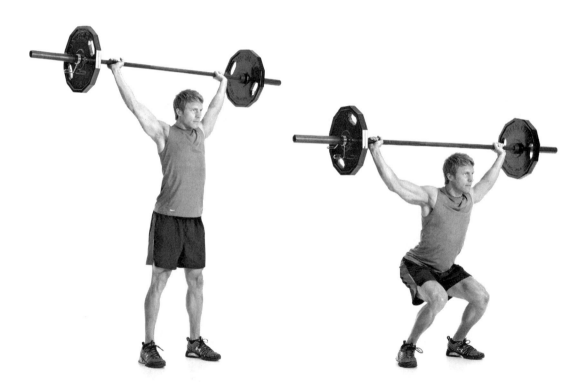

BULGARIAN SPLIT SQUAT

With the barbell on your shoulders and behind your neck, elevate your rear foot up onto a bench and split your front foot well out in front of you. Maintain an erect torso and descend into a deep squat, trying to get your rear knee close to the floor. Think of pushing through your heel during this movement. Complete all of your repetitions and then switch legs.

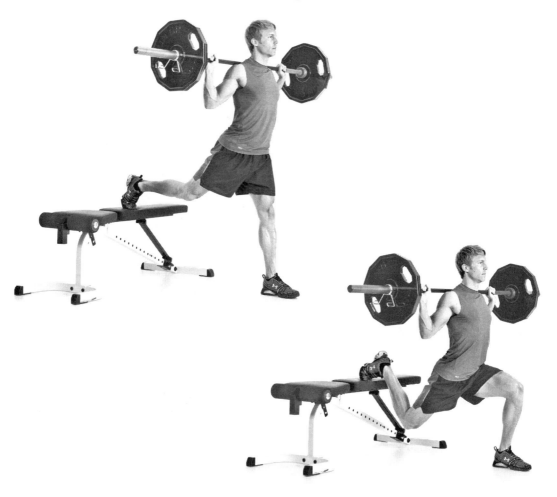

DROP LUNGE

Place the bar on your shoulders (behind your neck) with your feet close together. Drop one leg back and across behind your body while bending the front leg to get as low as possible. Drive back up to the start position to repeat on the other side. One repetition on each side is 1 full repetition. Be sure to keep the shoulders square and front foot pointed forward the whole time while letting your hips do the rotating.

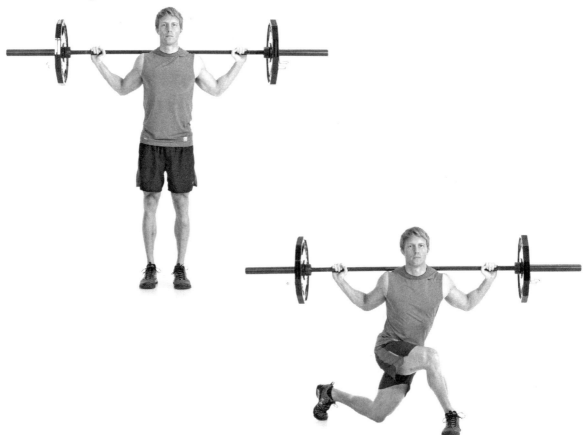

SINGLE-LEG SQUAT

Standing on top of a bench or a box, hang one foot off the side while reaching your arms forward. Descend into as deep a squat as possible by leaning forward and pushing your hips back and heel flat. Holding a small weight will help facilitate more balance and allow for a deeper squat. Learn how to gradually make this exercise more difficult once you are able to complete deep squats on all of your reps.

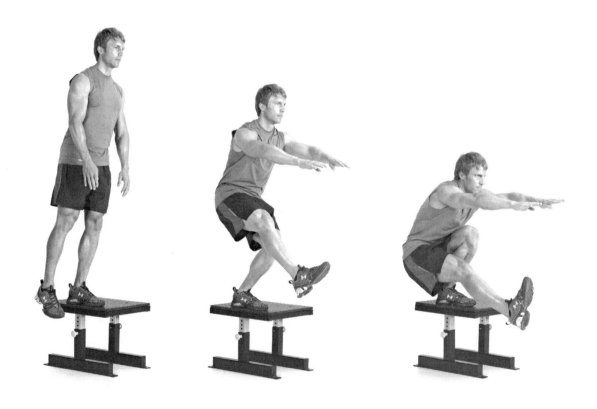

SPLIT SQUAT

Start with the bar behind your neck and feet wide with toes slightly pointed out. Push your hips back, lean forward, and laterally squat toward one side. Keep your heel flat in your deep squat as your back leg straightens out. Move back to the start position and then repeat on the other side.

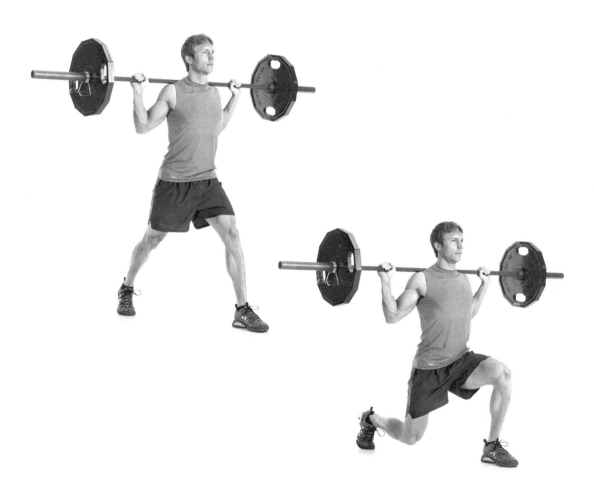

BENCH PRESS

Using either dumbbells or a barbell, perform a standard flat bench press using full range of motion.

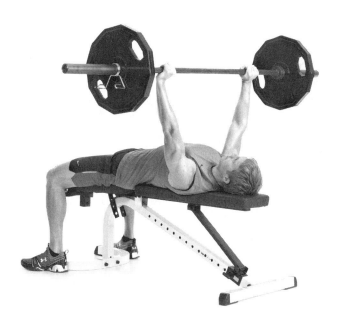

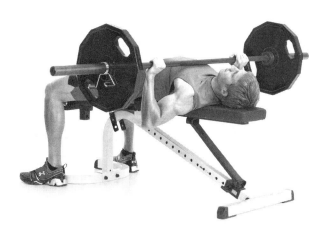

INCLINE PRESS

Using either dumbbells or a barbell, perform a standard incline bench press at approximately a 30-degree angle.

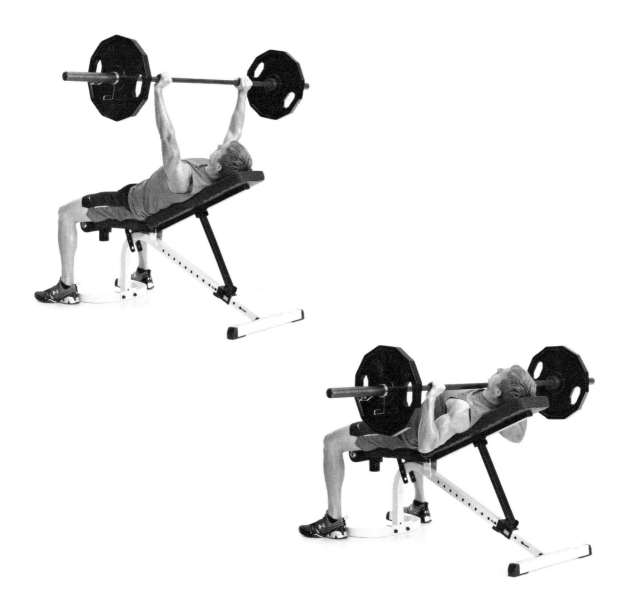

DUMBBELL ALTERNATING BENCH PRESS

Using dumbbells on either a flat or incline bench position, press one dumbbell up as you simultaneously lower the opposite dumbbell. There should be one dumbbell moving up and one moving down at all times.

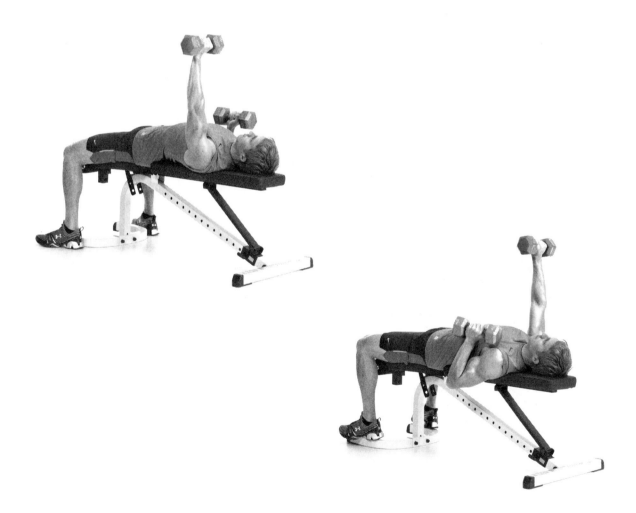

DUMBBELL HALF BENCH PRESS

Holding one dumbbell, position yourself on a bench so that half of your body is off the bench (the dumbbell side). You should have the dumbbell side's hip, shoulder, and head all halfway off the bench as you hold onto the bench near your head with the opposite arm. Push hard with the leg on the dumbbell side to keep the body flat and solid throughout the entire movement as you press the dumbbell.

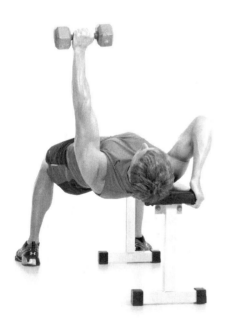
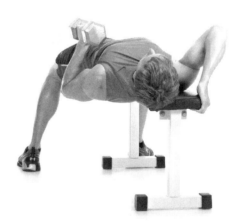

PUSH PRESS

Hold the weight at the shoulders, then dip and drive the weight upward. As the bar passes your face, drop your chin so that the weight finishes overhead and above your ears. Think of pushing the weight with your legs in this movement. You should extend your arms and legs at the same time as you press the weight overhead.

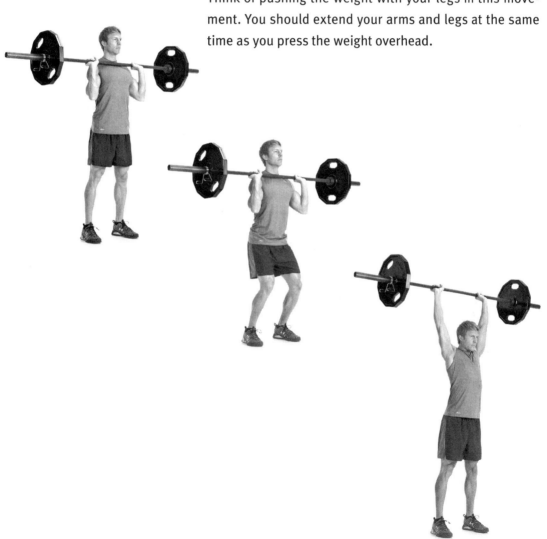

PUSH JERK

Hold the weight at your shoulders, then dip and drive the weight upward. As the bar passes your face, drop your chin so that the weight finishes overhead and above your ears. You should drop your hips and bend your knees as you extend your arms overhead.

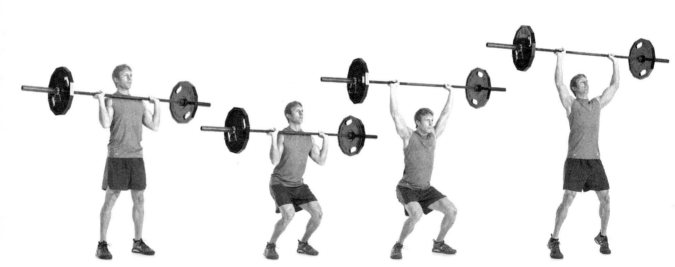

DUMBBELL PUSH PRESS

Holding one or two dumbbells, dip and drive the weight overhead using your legs. Your arms and legs should simultaneously extend as you press the weight overhead.

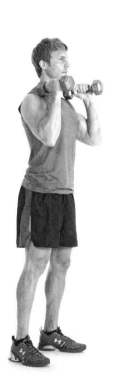
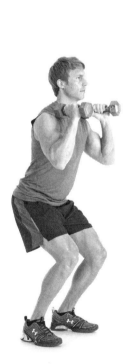
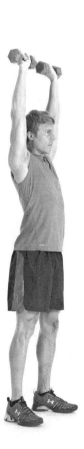

Dips

Using a shoulder-width grip on a dip station, lower yourself
as far as possible into the bottom position. Push up until
your arms are fully extended.

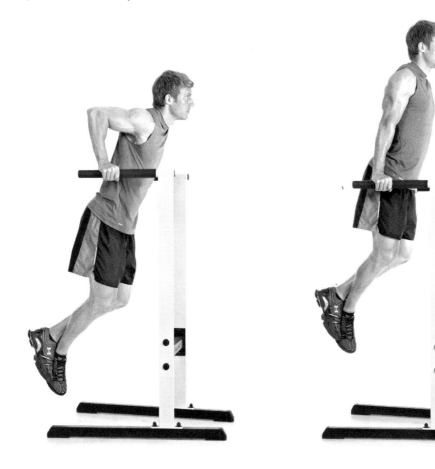

SUSPENDED PUSHUPS

Placing your feet into suspended rings, perform a pushup
as far as possible into the bottom position. Try to rotate
your hands so that they start with thumbs up at the top and
finish with thumbs pointed in at the bottom of the pushup.
You can make this exercise more difficult by elevating your
feet up onto a bench, a box, or even a stability ball.

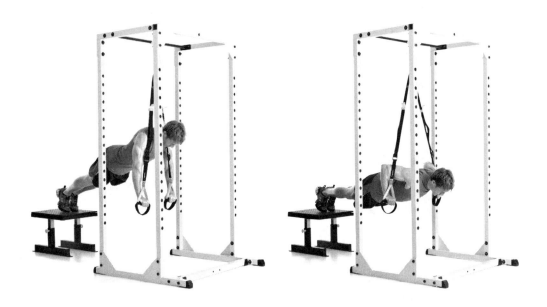

PULLUPS

Using a shoulder-width, pronated grip (palms facing away),
perform full-range-of-motion pullups, making sure to lower
to full extension of your arms for each repetition.

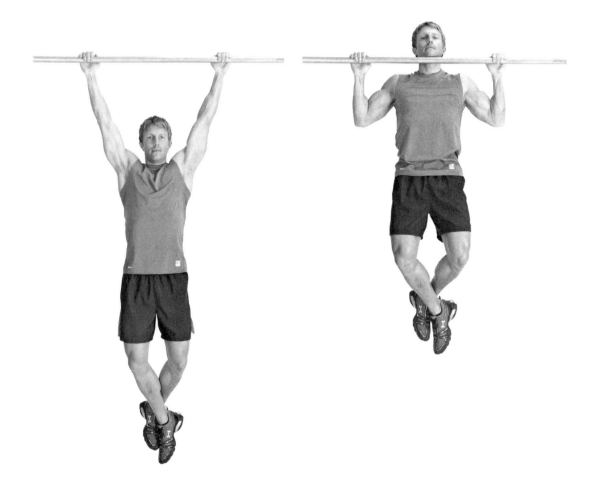

CHINUPS

Using a narrow, supinated grip (palms facing you), perform full-range-of-motion pullups, making sure to lower to full extension of your arms for each repetition.

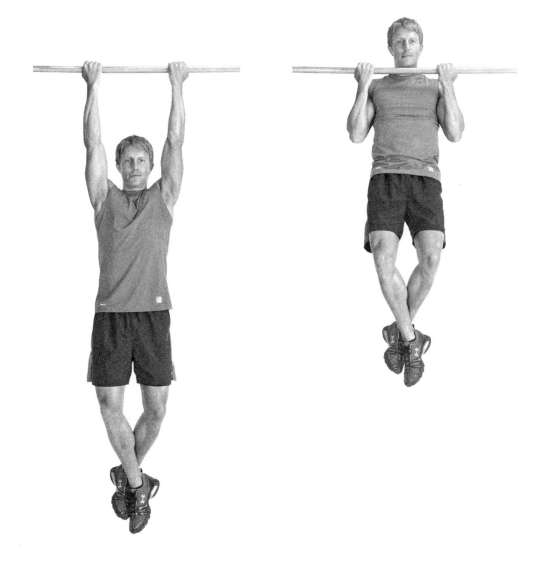

SIDE-TO-SIDE PULLUPS

Using a wider than shoulder-width pronated grip, perform
a pullup, attempting to pull your body toward one hand as
if you are trying to place your chin on that hand. Lower to
the bottom position and repeat on the other side. Each
pullup counts as 1 repetition.

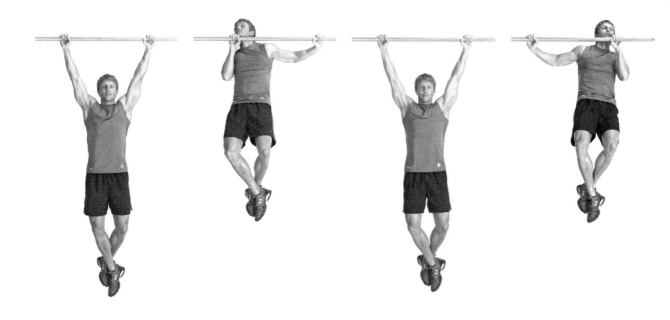

Horizontal pullups

Hanging underneath a bar with your legs straight and core tight, pull yourself up until your chest touches the bar. You can use any comfortable grip on this exercise. Elevate your feet to make this exercise more difficult.

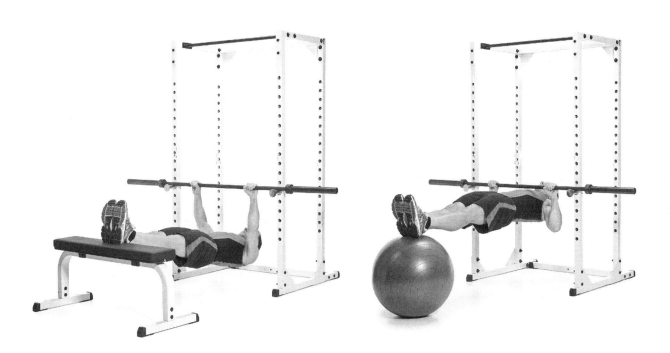

SUSPENDED ROWS

Hanging underneath suspended rings with your legs straight and core tight, pull yourself up as high as possible, trying to rotate your hands so that they start with your thumbs facing in and finish with your thumbs facing up at the top of the exercise. Elevate your feet to make this exercise more difficult.

ONE-ARM HORIZONTAL PULLUP

Hanging underneath a bar with one hand placed in the center of the bar and your legs slightly bent, pull up to the bar as you reach through with your opposite arm to facilitate the complete pull.

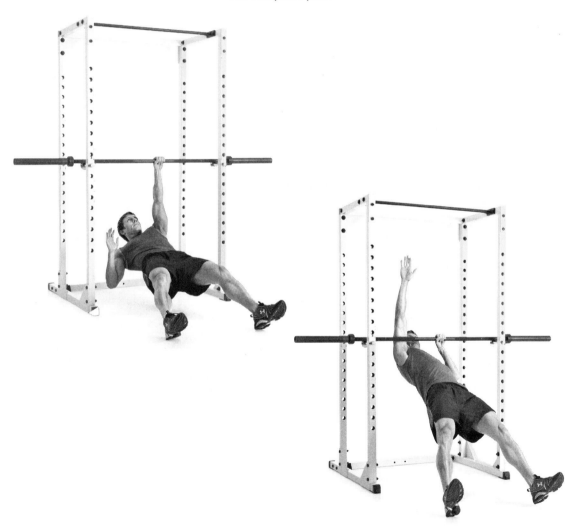

BENT-OVER ROW

Using a barbell or dumbbells, hold on to the weight in a bent-over position with your knees slightly bent and back flat. Row the weight up to your rib cage, making sure to stay in a strong bent-over position the entire time.

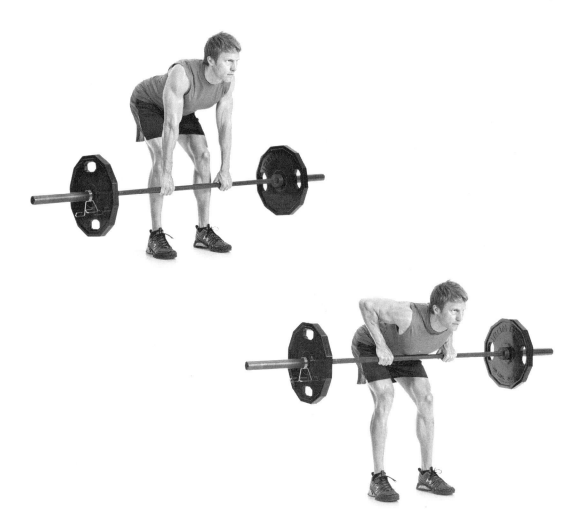

CABLE FACE PULLS

Using a rope attachment on a cable machine, set the pulley so that it starts slightly above your head. Stand tall with your core tight as you row the weight so that the pull finishes with your thumbs touching your temples or right near your ears. Make sure to use a full range of motion as you extend your arms back to the starting position, letting your shoulder blades stretch open.

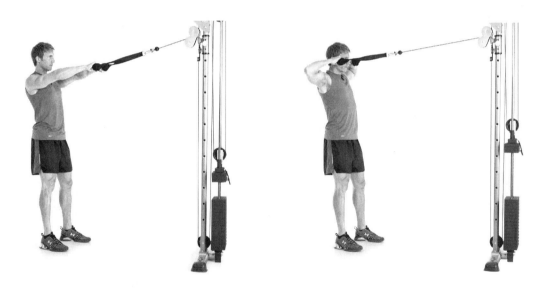

ONE-ARM DUMBBELL PLANK ROW

Position yourself using a bench so that you are holding a three-point plank position with one arm in the center of the bench right underneath your chest. Your body should be flat and solid as you hold a dumbbell in the other hand, letting it hang below you. Keeping your body rigid, row the weight up to your rib cage.

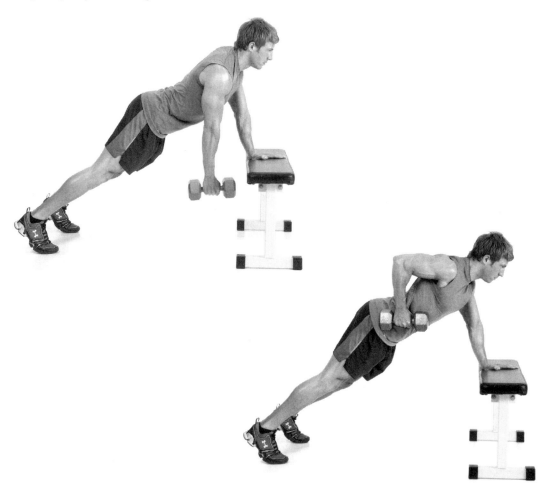

SPIDERMAN PUSHUPS

Using val slides or towels on a smooth floor surface, start in a pushup position. Slide your left arm out as far as possible, keeping that arm only slightly bent. As you reach out with this hand, bend your right arm to lower your body into a pushup position as you simultaneously bring your right knee to your left elbow.

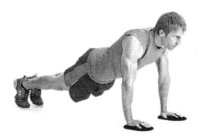

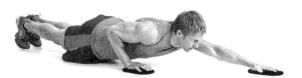

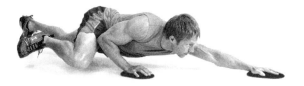

STANDING BARBELL ANTI-ROTATION

A barbell with a handle bar attachment works best on this exercise, but you can also perform this exercise without the attachment. Holding the bar high either on the handles or by grasping the end of the bar, keep your body tall and your core tight with your knees slightly bent. Let your arms rotate to one side as if you are trying to draw a large circle with the tip of the bar. Move as far as possible without letting your core collapse before repeating in the opposite direction.

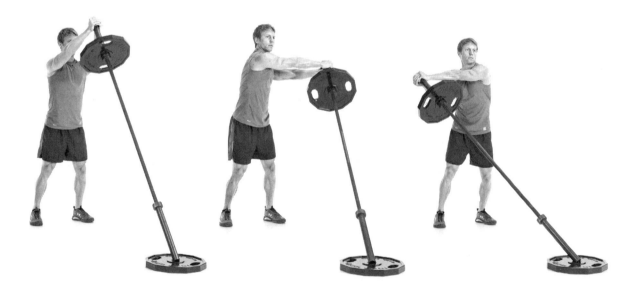

BARBELL SITUPS

Hold a barbell with a shoulder-width grip as you lie flat on the floor. Your legs will stay straight this entire movement. Push the bar forward as you sit up and pull the bar back over your head as you reach the midpoint. You should finish sitting tall with your legs straight and the bar above and behind your ears. Lower back to the starting position under control.

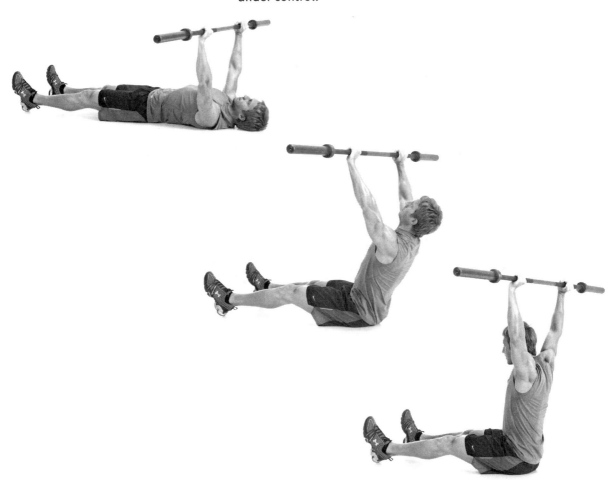

CABLE WOODCHOP (LOW TO HIGH)

Hold a single handle or rope attachment with both hands using a low cable position. Reach down so that your arms are fully extended and shoulders are facing the weight stack. Forcefully pull the load as you rotate your shoulders and turn your hips and shoulders away from the weight stack. Repeat on one side for specified number of reps; then switch to the opposite side. Be sure to pivot your back foot to facilitate as much range of motion as possible, and look up and reach to the ceiling at the end of the movement.

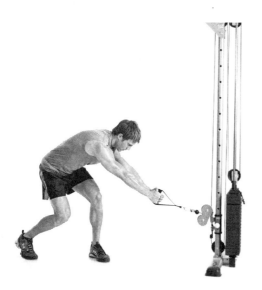
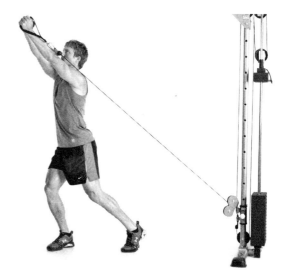

CABLE WOODCHOP (HIGH TO LOW)

Hold a single handle or rope attachment with both hands using a high cable position. Reach up so that your arms are fully extended and shoulders are facing the weight stack. Forcefully pull the load as you rotate your shoulders and turn your hips and shoulders away from the weight stack. Repeat on one side for specified number of reps; then switch to the opposite side. Be sure to pivot your back foot to facilitate as much range of motion as possible, and look down and reach to the floor at the end of the movement.

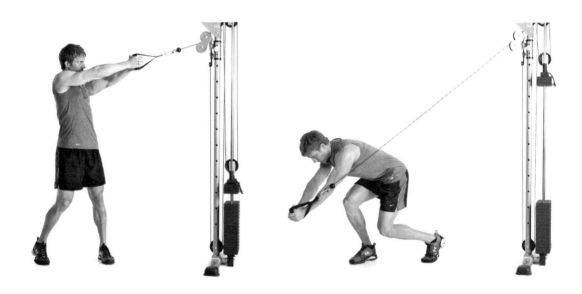

CABLE PUSH-PULL ANTI-ROTATION

Stand between two cable stacks or on a functional trainer with your feet even and torso tall and rigid. Holding one arm extended in front of you (to pull) and one arm at your chest (to press), simultaneously push and pull the cables while attempting to keep your body straight throughout the entire movement. The more weight you try to push and pull, the greater the core demands will be.

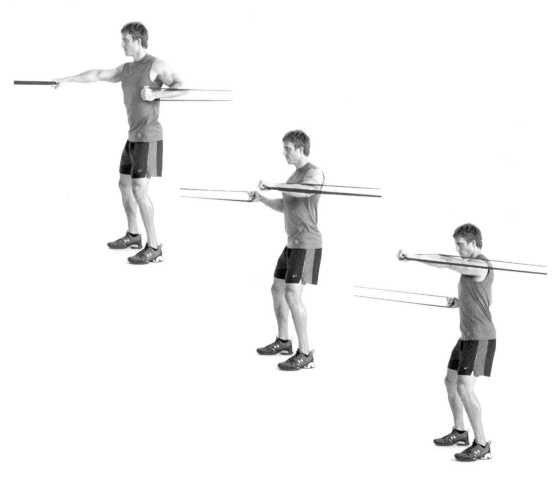

AB ROLLOUT

Hold a barbell at arm's length while on your knees. Push the bar out by leading with your arms and then following with your hips until you have pushed out as far as possible. Move back to the start position by leading with your hips, then finishing with your arms.

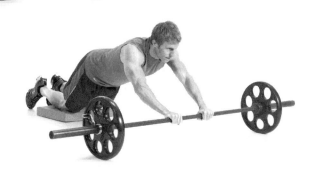

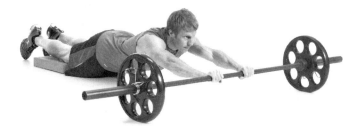

WINDMILLS

Hold a dumbbell or kettlebell overhead with your feet a little wider than shoulder-width apart and your knees almost completely locked out. Push your hips back and sideways (to the side of the kettlebell) while looking at the weight overhead and reach down to touch the floor between your feet. Perform all repetitions on that side before moving to the other side.

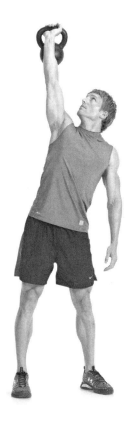
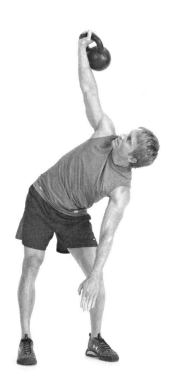
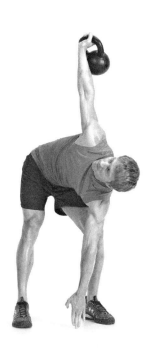

ROMANIAN DEADLIFT

Hold the bar using a shoulder-width grip and palms facing your body. With your knees slightly bent, push your hips back while keeping your chest up and your back flat, then lower the weight as far as possible. Think of reaching your chest forward rather than bending over to lower the weight.

GOOD MORNING

With the bar high on your shoulders and feet hip-width apart, pull your shoulders back and keep your lower back slightly arched or flat. Bend your knees slightly and hold them in this position throughout the set. Begin the movement by pushing your hips back as your shoulders move forward, then descend as far as possible while keeping your eyes up and your back flat.

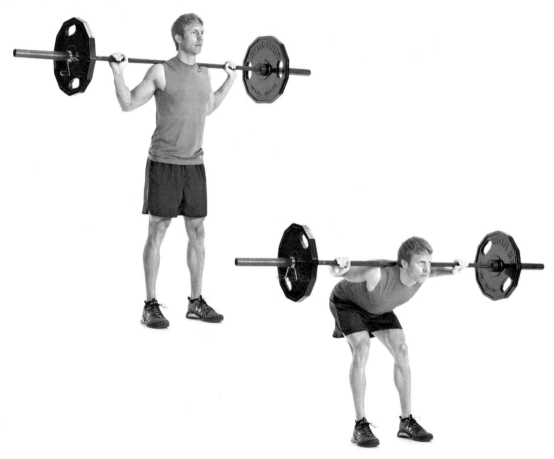

ONE-LEG BACK EXTENSION

Position yourself on a back extension bench, placing only one leg in the foothold. Keeping that leg straight, attempt to bend your knee as you are performing your back extensions, as this will help alleviate some of the pressure on your knee joint.

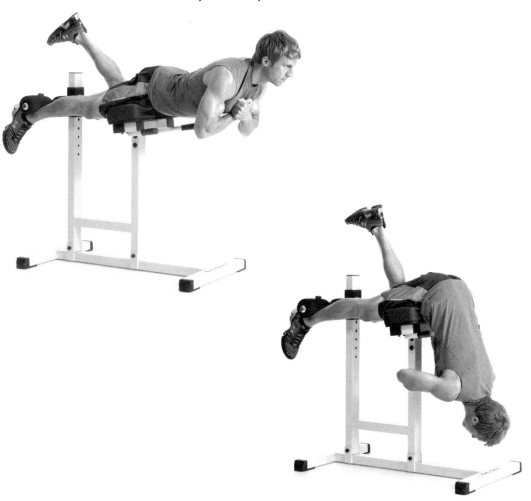

DUMBBELL ONE-LEG ROMANIAN DEADLIFT

Hold a dumbbell in one hand as you balance on the opposite foot. Lower the dumbbell down to that foot as you push your hips back with your knee slightly bent. Attempt to balance on that foot for all the repetitions, then switch legs and dumbbell to repeat on the other side.

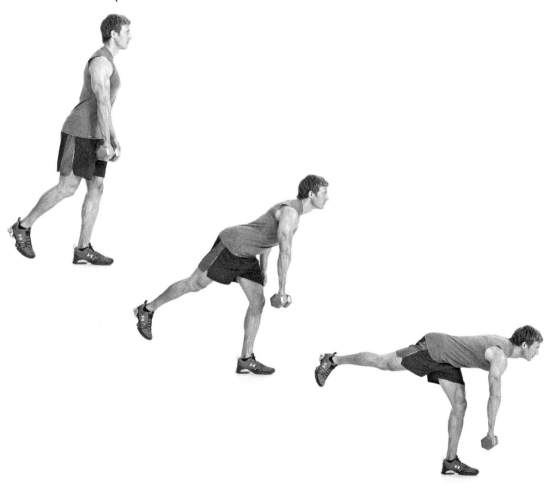

SEATED GOOD MORNING

Sit on a bench with a barbell behind your neck with your eyes up and lower back arched. Straighten your legs and place them out in front of you. Lower your chest toward the bench as far as possible as you keep your chest tall and eyes up. Do not let your lower back round during this movement.

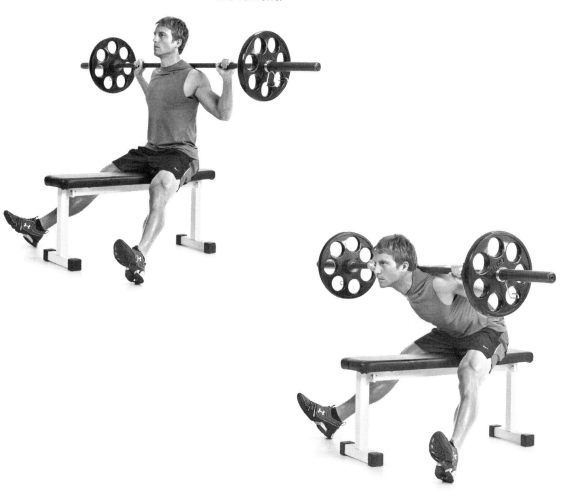

STABILITY BALL LEG CURL

Lie on your back on the floor with your legs up on top of a stability ball so that your calves are touching the ball. Raise your hips so that your body is straight, then curl the ball back toward you by digging your feet into the ball, bending your knees, and continuing to raise your hips. Slowly extend your legs back to the starting position, finishing by lowering your hips back to the floor. You can make this exercise more difficult by performing it with one leg.

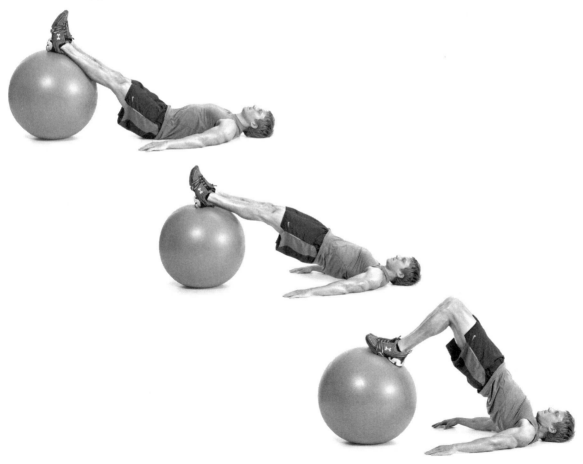

VAL SLIDE LEG CURL

Using a val slide under each foot or a towel on a smooth surface, lie on your back with a rolled-up towel under your hips if necessary. With your legs straight, pick your hips up so that they are off the towel and pull your feet back toward the towel. Your knees will bend and your hips will continue to rise as your feet curl in. This is a more difficult exercise than the stability ball leg curl. You can make this exercise even more difficult by performing it with one leg.

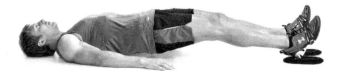

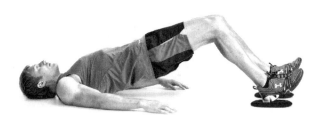

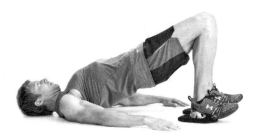

TIMED SET USING 30-SECOND WORK TO 60-SECOND REST INTERVALS	
SAMPLE CIRCUIT #1—BEGINNER	**SAMPLE CIRCUIT #2—ADVANCED**
1. Reverse lunge	1. Split squat (pause 3 seconds at bottom)
2. Pushup	2. Other leg forward
3. Plank walkup	3. Pushup (pause 3 seconds at bottom)
4. Split squat jump	4. Plank with weight transfer
	5. Squat jump (pause 3 seconds at bottom)

REVERSE LUNGE

Standing tall with feet together, reach back with one leg as far as possible as you bend the front leg, keeping your torso tall. Push back up to the start position, then repeat on the other leg. One repetition is both right and left legs.

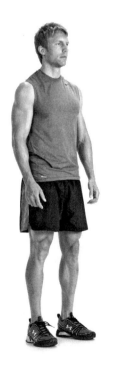
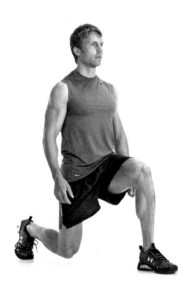
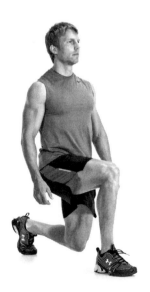

PLANK WALKUP

Position yourself in a plank/bridge position on elbows and toes. Push yourself up to a pushup position, attempting to minimize body movement. Pause at the top, then lower back to the plank position. Change your lead arm to the pushup position on each pushup.

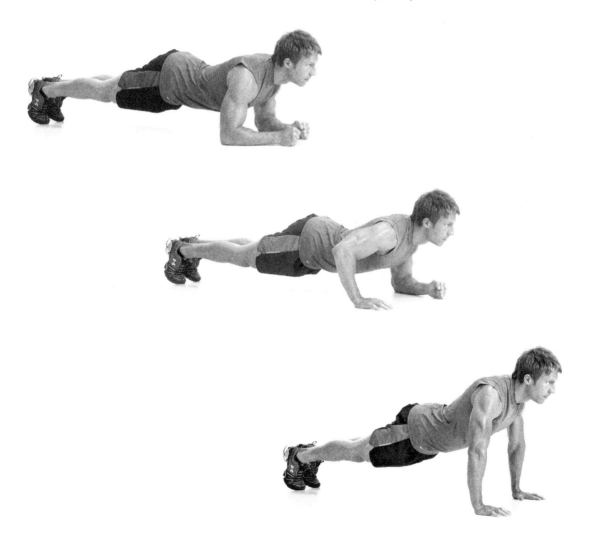

SPLIT SQUAT JUMP

Start with your feet split with one leg forward and one leg back. Lower into a deep squat, then explode upward, switching your legs in midair. Repeat on the other side.

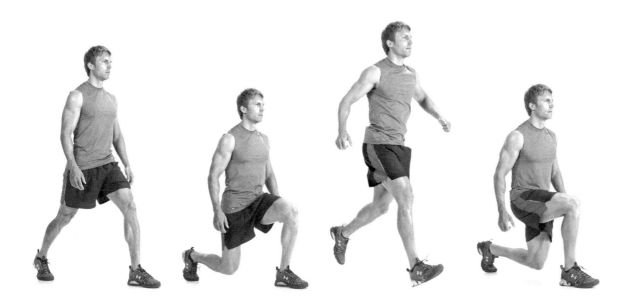

PLANK WITH WEIGHT TRANSFER

Start in a solid plank/bridge position on elbows and toes with a small weight set outside one of your arms. Without too much body movement, pick up the weight with the close hand and transfer it to the other hand. Reach out and place the weight far outside with the opposite hand. Pause and then repeat by transferring the weight back to the other side.

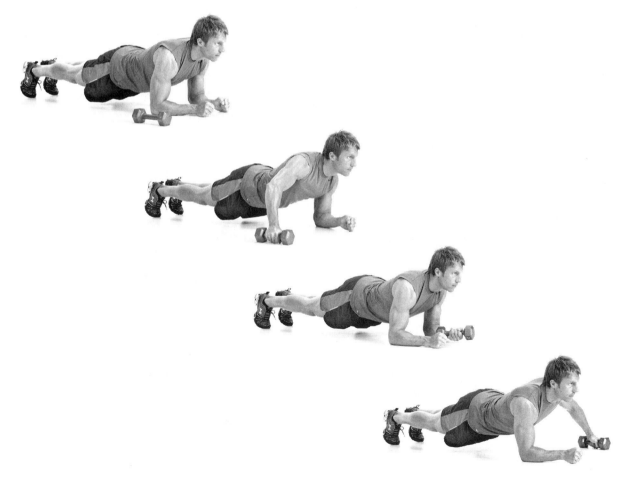

COACH DOS'S FAVORITE 30/30 INTERVAL EXERCISE LIST		
KETTLEBELL	**BARBELL**	**BODY WEIGHT**
Alternating swings	Jump shrug	Burpees
Snatch (each arm)	Push press	Alternating lunges
Windmill (each side)	Good morning	Pushups
Front squat (each side)	Bent-over row	Mountain climbers
Push press (each arm)	Front squats	Squat jumps
Sumo jump squat		
10 minutes = one time through	10 minutes = two times through	10 minutes = two times through
20 minutes = two times through	20 minutes = four times through	20 minutes = four times through

KETTLEBELL FRONT SQUAT (ONE SIDED)

Hold a single kettlebell in at the shoulder in the clean catch position and squat as deep as possible. Use the other arm to help offset the load in any way. Try to stay tall and not lean toward the weight during the movement. This is a tremendous core exercise as well.

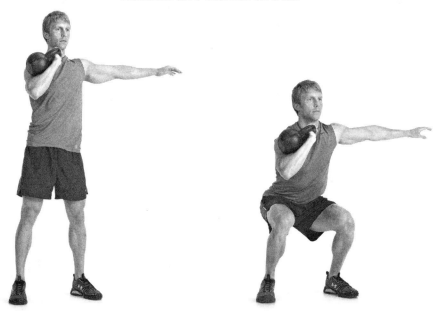

KETTLEBELL SUMO JUMP SQUAT

Hold the kettlebell in front of you at arm's length with feet in the wide sumo-style base. Lower the weight to the floor as you bend your knees and lower your hips with your torso tall. Explode up off the ground and absorb the load all the way back down to repeat for your next repetition.

TIMED SETS WITH 40 SECONDS WORK: 20 SECONDS REST

SAMPLE #1	SAMPLE #2	SAMPLE #3
Val slide atomic pushup	TRX atomic pushup	Medicine ball split lunge jump
Kettlebell swing	TRX wakeboard jump	Medicine ball pushup
Val slide ab slide	TRX rows	Medicine ball st leg situp
Kettlebell alternate swing	TRX one-leg squat jumps	Medicine ball overhead squat
Val slide sled push	TRX superman	Medicine ball burpees

VAL SLIDE ATOMIC PUSHUP

With your feet on val slides, perform a pushup; but as you come up to the top of the movement, pull the knees into your stomach as your feet slide in to your chest then back out for the next pushup.

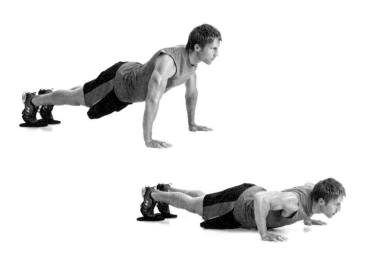

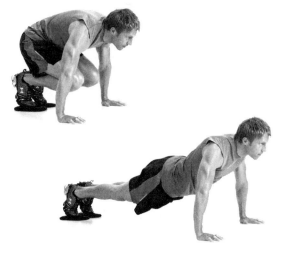

KETTLEBELL SWING

Hold the kettlebell in one hand and lower to the power position with your shoulders forward, hips back, and forearm in contact with your inner thigh. Swing the dumbbell using your hip extension to drive the weight up. At the highest point of the swing, the weight will feel weightless; immediately decelerate the weight back to the starting position with the other arm. One repetition is a swing with both arms.

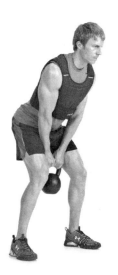
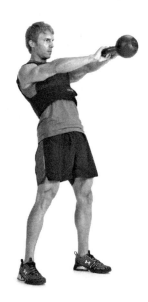

VAL SLIDE AB SLIDE

Starting on your knees with your hands on the val slides, push your hips forward as you slide your hands out as far as possible before pulling back to the start position.

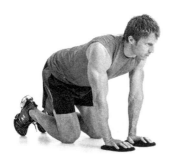

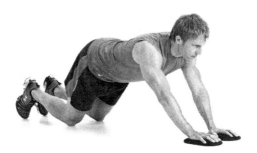

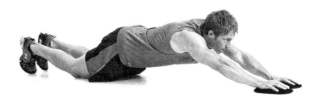

KETTLEBELL ALTERNATING SWING

Place the kettlebell between your feet. To get in the starting position, push your butt back and look straight ahead. Clean the kettlebell to your shoulder. Drop the kettlebell to a hanging position between your legs while keeping your hamstrings loaded.

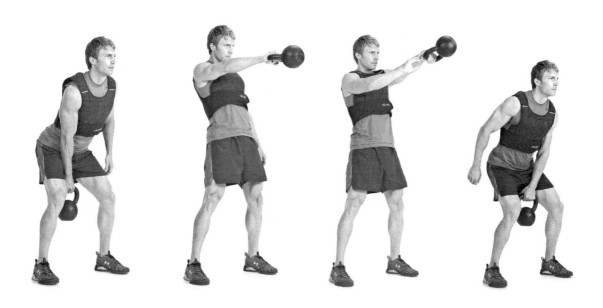

VAL SLIDE SLED PUSH

With your hands on the val slides, keep your hips low as you push the slides around a smooth floor surface for the duration of the interval.

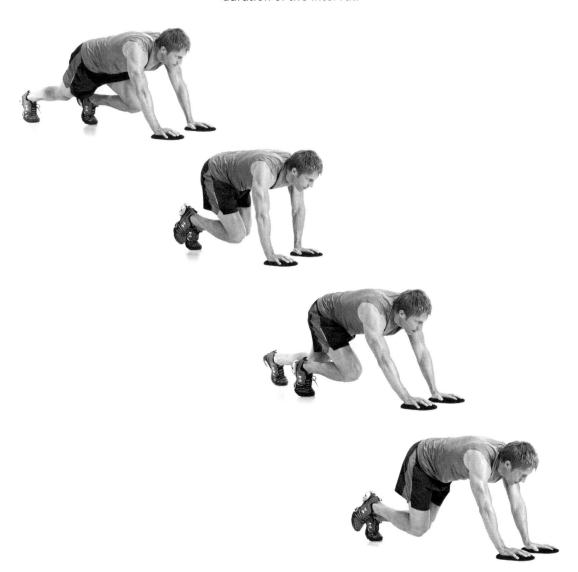

TRX ATOMIC PUSHUP

With your feet in the TRX foot straps, perform a pushup; but as you reach the top of the movement, pull the knees in toward your stomach then push them back out for the next repetition.

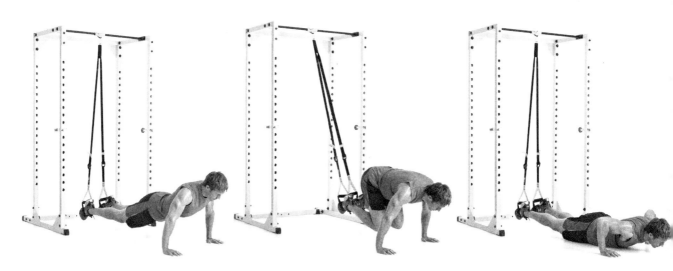

TRX 180 DEGREE JUMPS

Start with your hips turned perpendicular to your shoulders with rear foot crossed over so that it starts in front of front foot. Keep your feet wider than shoulder width apart. Keep your eyes and shoulders facing forward the entire time; jump as high as possible rotating your hips 180 degrees in the opposite direction at the highest point. Land with your rear foot crossed over in front of your front foot.

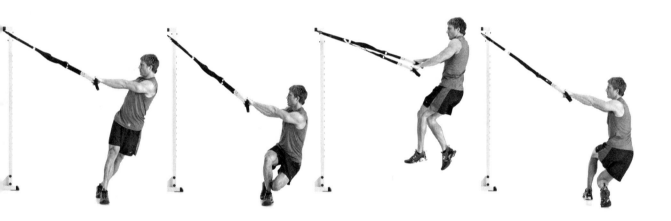

TRX ROWS

Start with one foot placed in front of your body with your opposite leg extended out in front of you. Squat deep with your arms extended; jump as high as possible switching legs at the high point of the jump, landing on the opposite foot. Use your arms for stabilizing and decelerating as needed.

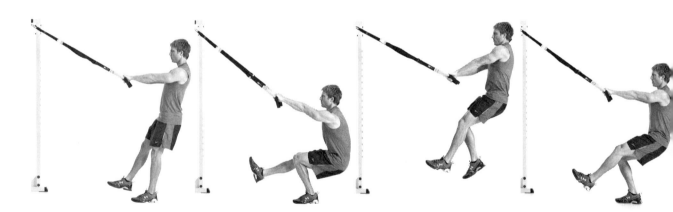

TRX SUPERMAN

Get in a pushup position with your hands in TRX handles. Reach your arms out as far as possible, then return to the starting position. (You can make this move more difficult by lowering the handles and/or elevating your feet on something stable like a bench or box.)

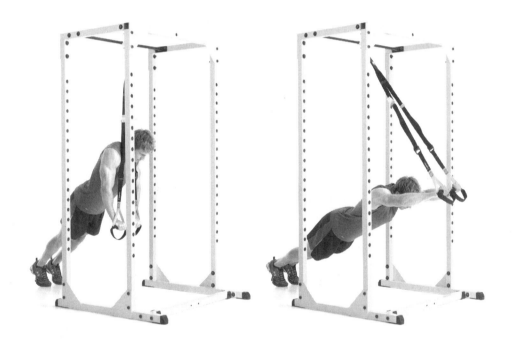

MEDICINE BALL SPLIT JUMP

Holding the medicine ball close to your chest with both arms and feet split wide in a forward and backward stance, jump as high as possible, switching legs in the air.

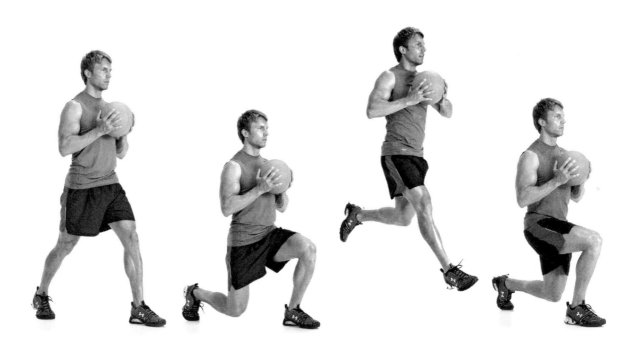

MEDICINE BALL PUSHUP

Start with one hand on a medicine ball and one hand on the floor. Perform a pushup and forcefully push yourself up and over the top of the ball so that you land with the opposite hand on the ball and the other hand on the floor.

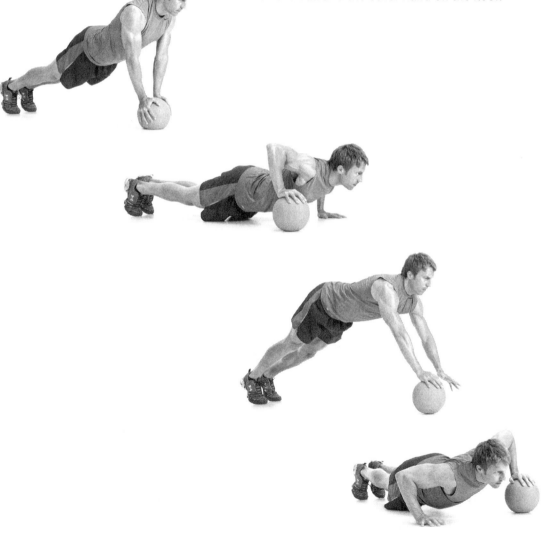

MEDICINE BALL STRAIGHT LEG SITUP

Lie on your back with your legs straight, holding a medicine ball over your chest with your arms extended. Push the ball slightly forward as you sit up with your shoulders tall and your chest out. Finish with the ball directly over the top of your head.

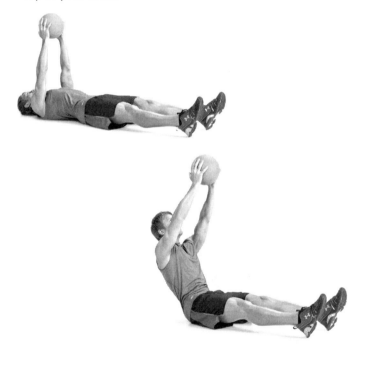

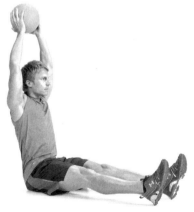

MEDICINE BALL OVERHEAD SQUAT

With your feet in a squatting base and holding a medicine ball directly over your head with your arms extended, squat as deep as possible. Try to keep the ball over your head without moving it forward too much.

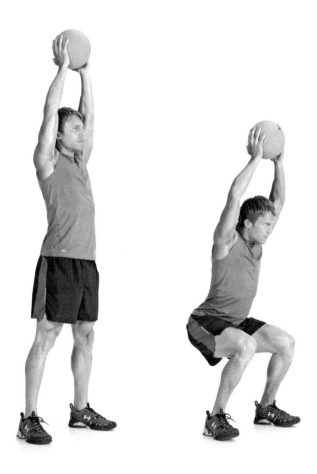

MEDICINE BALL BURPEE

Standing with a medicine ball in front of you at arms length; squat down placing the ball on the floor as you kick your legs back into a pushup position, using the ball as your base. Quickly reverse this movement and jump your legs back into a squatting position; then forcefully jump as you reach the medicine ball as high overhead as possible.

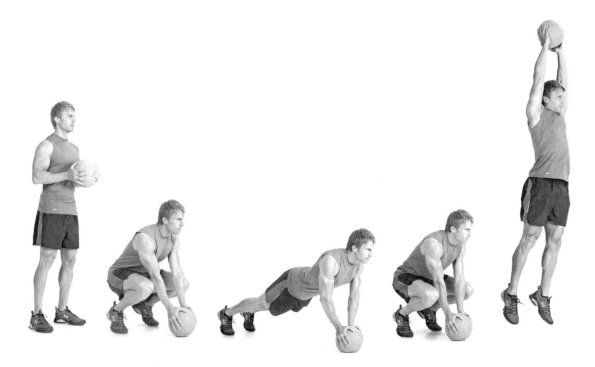

TWO-HANDED SWING

Holding the kettlebell with both hands and in a squat-type base, bend your knees and move your shoulders forward so that your forearms are in contact with your inner thighs. Drive the weight upward and out using the extension of your hips to move the load. Decelerate the load back to the starting position.

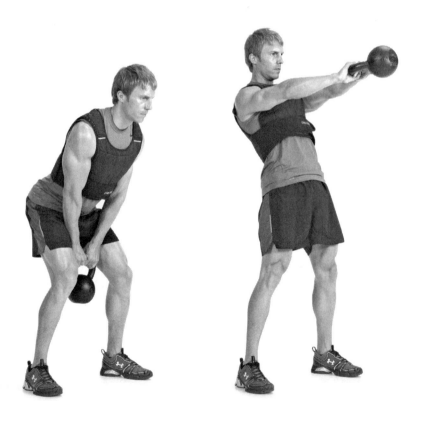

FRONT SQUAT + PUSH PRESS

This is a hybrid movement starting with the barbell being held at the shoulders. Descend into a deep front squat. As you raise up and near the top of the squat, explode the weight overhead (do a push press). As you lower the bar back down, you should automatically start descending into your next squat.

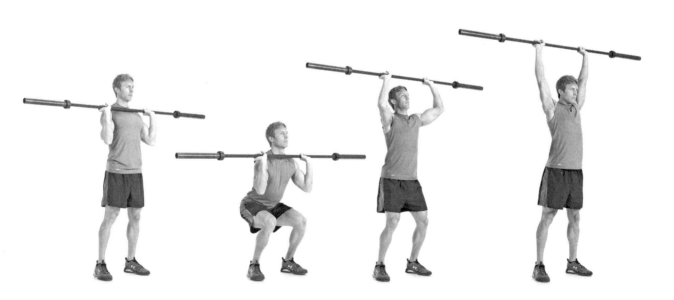

SUMO SQUAT + CURL AND PRESS

This is also a hybrid movement. Stand with your feet in the side sumo base position, holding a dumbbell in each hand and hanging at arm's length in front of you. Lower down until the dumbbells touch the floor. As you ascend from the squat, immediately begin curling the weights to your shoulders and then explode them overhead as you near the top of the squat (do a push press). Reverse all the movements to bring the dumbbells back down and into your next squat.

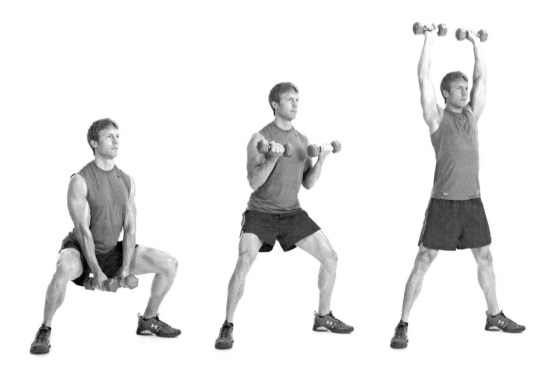

7

TABATA PROTOCOL

There I stood, stopwatch in hand, ready for my first experience with the infamous Tabata Protocol. My plan: Perform squat jumps as fast and furious as I could for 20 seconds, rest for 10 seconds, and do this for a total of eight rounds . . . a paltry 4 minutes of my life. "No problem" I told myself, and off I went. Round number one wasn't so bad; I completed almost 20 squat jumps and my confidence was building. After round number two, however, whatever confidence I had was fading, my number of squat jumps started to decrease, and my heart rate was doing the opposite. My legs were burning, the 10-second rest periods seemed like the blink of an eye, and my heart felt like it was trying to burst out of my throat. Finally, I finished my eighth interval and crashed to the floor, huffing and puffing, as folks in my gym looked over at me, checking to see if I might need medical attention.

LET'S GET SOMETHING STRAIGHT HERE

The Tabata Protocol is perhaps the most bastardized form of exercise ever. People have gleaned some insight into the research findings and decided to put their own little spin on this highly effective protocol. Most of these spin-offs have resulted in an easier, happier form of this protocol. People performing squats, pushups, or lunges at a leisurely pace and telling their friends they just performed some Tabatas in the gym are not being honest. Sorry folks, but these *are not* Tabatas—at least not what the researchers meant for the world to turn their protocol into.

Let's go back to the research for a second. The Tabata Protocol subjects performed six to eight rounds of this all-out effort in the study. Yes, some of the subjects never even made it through the protocol's eight rounds or 4 minutes of work! If this doesn't tell you

191

how hard they were working, I don't know what would. All-out effort means just that—working as hard as you can for the entire interval period. The true key to this protocol and to its benefits is the concept of maximum intensity and *not* pacing. This type of intensity is necessary if you want to reap the benefits found in the research study.

WHAT IF I JUST CAN'T MAKE IT THROUGH AN ALL-OUT TABATA?

No problem, as this is where my simple modifications and progressions will help you. Sure, some might say that I have therefore personally bastardized this great cardio method, but I think my modifications are more in line with the true intention of this protocol.

Step 1 in this progression is to perform eight rounds of this protocol using only a 10-second work and a 20-second rest interval. The time to completion is still 4 minutes, but the work is cut in half. I like this interval not only for beginners (since 10 seconds is a lot more realistic for a beginner), but also for certain types of activities like sprints and agilities, which I will talk about in the next chapter.

Step 2 is to perform eight rounds using 15-second work and rest intervals. You see that we are starting to creep toward the tra-

ditional Tabata, but the extra 5 seconds of rest coupled with the 5 fewer seconds of work still makes a huge difference and allows for increased intensity during your work intervals.

Step 3 is to perform the standard 20 seconds of work and 10 seconds of rest for the eight rounds. My recommendation is that if you are still experiencing big drops in repetitions and performance in the latter rounds of the standard Tabata, go back to the step 1 15/15 intervals and continue to push your intensity. I have seen people perform exercises like burpees and complete 10 in the first round, then have their work deteriorate to two or three in the latter rounds, but this is not what we are looking for in this protocol.

COACH DOS'S FAVORITE TABATAS

I have lots of favorite exercise movements for Tabatas. Here are a few:

TABATA EXERCISE EXAMPLES
Jump rope (fast!)
Hitting or kicking a heavy bag
Burpees
Kettlebell swings
Squat jumps
Split squat jumps
Speed jumps
Plyo pushups
Mountain climbers

These are all easy movements that can be performed quickly and in a small area. Many of these movements can also be combined in an alternating fashion so that we don't get too much muscular fatigue in one specific area. For example, alternating squat jumps and mountain climbers or plyometric pushups will help offset the muscular fatigue in the legs compared to if you just did the squat jumps the entire time.

Below I have listed my very favorite exercise sequences for each time period of Tabatas.

In Chapter 9 I will talk about a few other tools that we can use to perform our Tabatas, along with other timed set-style circuits. The possibilities are virtually endless, so take advantage of all these new tools in your cardio strength toolbox. As with the 30/30 intervals, my friends at coachdosmusic.com have created some custom Coach Dos Tabata tracks that you can download for free.

10-SECOND WORK TO 20-SECOND REST INTERVALS	15-SECOND WORK TO 15-SECOND REST INTERVALS	20-SECOND WORK TO 10-SECOND REST INTERVALS
Dumbbell burpees	Medicine ball / Plyo pushups	Jump rope
Squat and press	Medicine ball / Squat jumps	Burpees
Repeat in alternating fashion	Medicine ball / Mountain climbers	*Repeat in alternating fashion*
	Medicine ball / Split squat jumps	
	Repeat all four exercises	

JUMP ROPE

Pick the pattern that you are most efficient in and go as fast and as hard as possible.

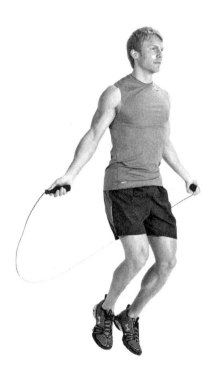

HITTING OR KICKING A HEAVY BAG

Just like it sounds. Use any kicking or punching patterns or combinations and go 100 percent for the time period.

SPEED JUMPS

These are similar to squat jumps, but you only lower into about a one-quarter squat. The goal here is maximum rep-etitions and minimal floor contact time.

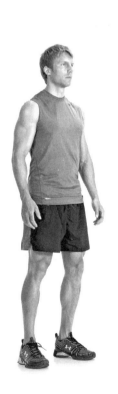
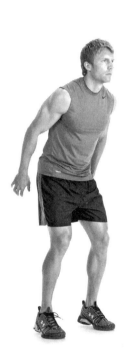
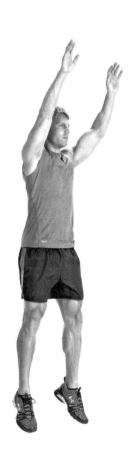

MEDICINE BALL / PLYO PUSHUPS

Place one hand on a medicine ball and one on the floor. Explode up and across, landing on the other side of the ball with your opposite hand on the ball. Repeat and explode back across on your next repetition.

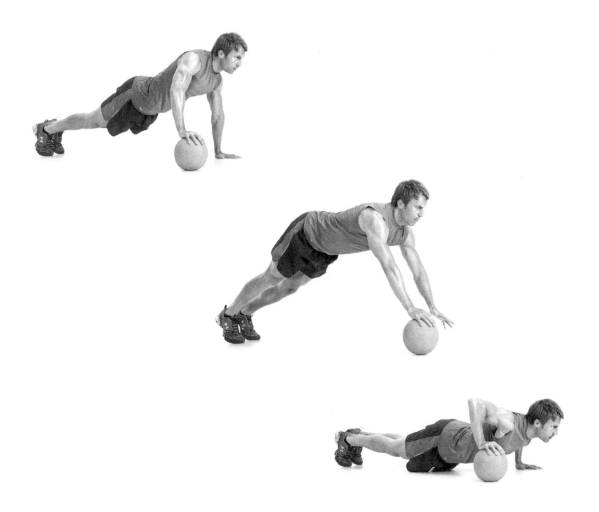

MEDICINE BALL / SQUAT JUMPS

These are just traditional squat jumps while holding the medicine ball close to your chest.

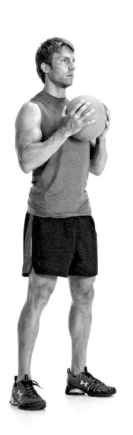
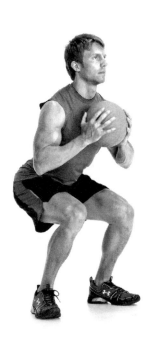
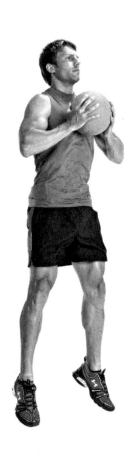

MEDICINE BALL / MOUNTAIN CLIMBERS

These are traditional mountain climbers, only with your hands on the ball. This is a more difficult version since the ball has a tendency to move, thus creating more core demands.

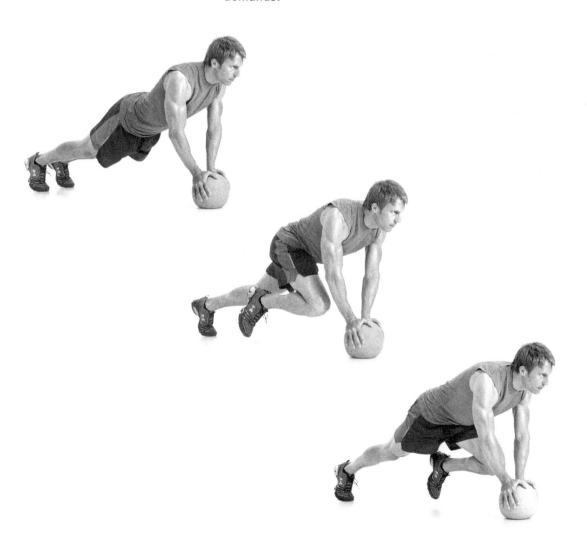

MEDICINE BALL / SPLIT SQUAT JUMPS

These are traditional split squat jumps while holding the medicine ball across your chest.

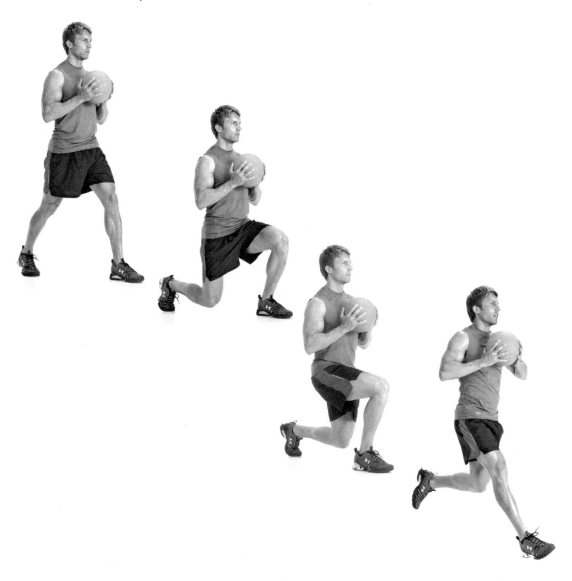

THE GREAT OUTDOORS

One of the most fun things I do in my own training regimen is get out of the gym and exercise outside in our great Southern California weather. I know, I know, some of you folks live in areas that don't see a lot of sunshine. Regardless, it's great to change up the scenery once in a while; if it's not outdoors, maybe it's in a basketball gym or on an indoor track. Boredom and the same old routine can often result in stagnant workouts and decreased progress, so take a chance and try some of these great cardio strength options outside of the gym.

SPRINT TRAINING

Anyone who has ever incorporated sprint training into his conditioning programs will attest to one thing: NOTHING seems to elicit the feeling that you get the day after. Even avid runners often talk about the huge differences they feel after incorporating sprint

training. In my everyday conditioning of our athletic teams, we utilize a large array of sprint intervals when performing our sport-specific energy system training. These intervals range from very-high-intensity, short sprints with longer rest intervals to longer, less intense sprints with relatively shorter rest intervals.

AEROBIC VERSUS ANAEROBIC SPRINT INTERVALS

I often hear people tell me that they have been doing "sprint intervals." Upon further examination, these folks are usually doing more of a modified aerobic interval run. Let me explain. When you think of sprinting, think of all-out running. Think about what you need to do after sprinting all out for, say, 15 to 20 seconds—most likely you will need to stop to gather yourself and recover before doing it again, right? Many times when people describe their "sprint intervals," they tell me they did 20 minutes on a treadmill, sprinting for 60 seconds, and then jogging for 60 seconds, etc. I will argue that very few of us are actually able to sprint for anywhere close to 60 seconds and, if we were able to, we wouldn't be able to jog during the rest interval. What these people are describing is more of an aerobic interval, a pacing where you run hard almost to your anaerobic threshold, then back off to a tolerable pace to recover. There is nothing wrong with this type of interval training; in fact, it is a great progression to lead you into the higher intensity, true sprint intervals that await you.

DECIDING ON WORK-TO-REST RATIOS

To begin, we want to establish some general "rules" when performing sprint intervals. Creating the optimal work-to-rest ratio will depend on two main factors: the intensity and the duration of the work interval. The greater the intensity and the shorter the work interval (usually these go hand in hand), the greater the work-to-rest ratio will be. The longer and less intense the work interval, the smaller the work-to-rest ratio will be. For example, something like a 40-yard sprint would be best suited to around a 1:4 work-to-rest ratio. This means that if it takes you 6 seconds to run this distance, you would rest 24 seconds. This sort of ratio allows for adequate recovery so that you can push hard enough on the next repetition. On the other hand, something like a 100-yard sprint might take you somewhere between 15 to 18 seconds to complete. In this case, you might only need a 1:2 ratio, resulting in a 30- to 36-second rest interval. Below is a layout of several distances with approximate completion times, along with the prescribed work-to-rest ratios. Also listed are some approximate sprint times, along with prescribed work-to-rest ratios. Keep in mind

SPRINT DISTANCES AND WORK:REST RATIOS

DISTANCE	10–20 YARDS	30–40 YARDS	60–80 YARDS	100–110 YARDS	HALF GASSER*	200 YARDS	400 YARDS
Approximate time to complete	2–3 seconds	4–6 seconds	9–12 seconds	15–20 seconds	17–22 seconds	35–45 seconds	75–95 seconds
Work:rest	1:5–6	1:4–5	1:3	1:2	1:2	1:2	1:2
Approximate rest times	10–18 seconds	16–30 seconds	27–36 seconds	30–40 seconds	34–44 seconds	70–90 seconds	150–190 seconds

*Half gasser is a sprint for 50 yards, then a turnaround and sprint back 50 yards

SAMPLE SPRINT WORKOUTS

DISTANCE	REPETITIONS	WORK:REST RATIO	APPROXIMATE TOTAL WORK TIME	APPROXIMATE TOTAL REST TIME	TOTAL WORKOUT TIME
Half Gasser	10	1:2	3½ minutes	6 minutes	9–10 minutes
80 yards & 60 yards	8 repetitions at 80 yards 6 repetitions at 60 yards	1:3	3 minutes	5½ minutes	8–9 minutes
20 yards	20	1:5–6	1–½ minutes	6–8 minutes	7–10 minutes

*Half gasser is a sprint for 50 yards, then a turnaround and sprint back 50 yards

that these completion times are estimates and your needs will vary depending on your fitness level. Regardless, the ratios should stay the same.

Above are a few sample sprint workouts, along with their estimated completion times. Remember, don't be fooled by the brevity of the sessions. Just because you stop doesn't mean your body has stopped working!

AGILITY TRAINING

In my opinion, one of the most effective and intense forms of sprint training is change of direction or agility training. When we force our bodies to change direction, we are forcing it to repeatedly decelerate and accelerate. This process has an amazing effect on both our muscular and cardiovascular systems.

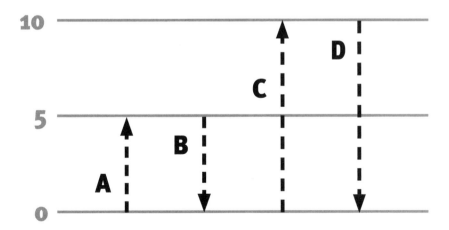

You are limited in most agility training drills only by your imagination, but most important is to think about your work-to-rest ratios once again. You can use the same ratios as in the prescribed sprint workouts, but keep in mind that many agility drills are relatively short in duration so you will be using the higher ratios for the most part. Here are two of my favorite simple agility drills.

Five and back/10 and backs—These are high-intensity changes of direction where you will sprint 5 yards, touch, turn, sprint back to the start, touch, turn, sprint 10 yards, touch, and sprint back to the start. Just follow the pattern shown on page 189, going from A to B to C to D. Average time to complete this drill is 9 to 12 seconds.

Pro Agility or 5/10/5 drill—This is a very popular agility test (shown below) used by many collegiate and professional teams. You start straddling the middle line, move to your right, touch at 5 yards with your right hand, turn, sprint back to your left for 10 yards, touch with your left hand, turn once more, and sprint back through your starting point. On your next repetition, start by moving to your left first. Average time to complete the drill is 5 to 7 seconds.

By seeing how long it takes to complete each drill, you can use the ratio guidelines already noted to determine how much rest you should take between work intervals. Keep in mind that when you are having to decelerate and stop and then re-accelerate, your intensity will tend to increase. Because of this you might want to increase the ratios just a little bit to facilitate this increase in work.

Here is a sample interval workout (opposite) using these two agility drills:

I recommend mixing both the sprint and the agility intervals each session to really

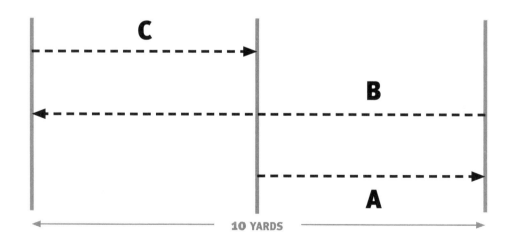

10 YARDS

SAMPLE AGILITY WORKOUT		
DRILL	**FIVE AND BACK/10 AND BACK**	**PRO AGILITY 5/10/5**
Repetitions	10	10
Work:rest ratio	1:3–4	1:5–6
Approximate total work time	1½–2 minutes	50–70 seconds
Approximate total rest time	4½–8 minutes	4–7 minutes
Total workout time	6–10 minutes	5–9 minutes

spice things up. Here's a sample mixed (advanced fitness level) workout, a simple workout that involves only approximately 4½ to 6 minutes of actual work and a total of about 14 to 19 minutes to complete. Like I said before, don't let the short duration fool you, though!

CHAOS AGILITY INTERVALS

CHAOS agility training is something my friend Jim Liston and I came up with years ago. It's nothing new, just something we noted that was not done nearly enough in sport performance speed training. Simply put, CHAOS drills are what we call "open" agility drills. These are drills that do not have a set distance before changing direction; these drills are driven by visual, verbal, or physical cues. For example, you may start running, then change direction when someone tells you, points, or touches you.

These CHAOS drills have all the benefits of the previously described agility drills but take them even a step further. The unpredictability causes us to decelerate and accelerate with even greater intensity, thus making these drills even more effective at causing that all-important metabolic disturbance we are seeking with cardio strength training. The simplest example of a CHAOS drill is to start side shuffling as fast as possible as someone randomly yells out "switch." Each time you hear "switch," you would change the direction of your shuffle. This shuffle can be replaced by a sprint, a backpedal, a carioca, a bear crawl, and so

DISTANCE	**HALF GASSER**	**PRO AGILITY 5/10/5**
Repetitions	10	10
Work:rest ratio	1:2	1:5–6
Approximate total work time	3½–4 minutes	50–70 seconds
Approximate total rest time	6 minutes	4–7 minutes
Total workout time	9–10 minutes	5–9 minutes

forth. For the most part, you would need a partner to perform these types of drills so he could either shout out or point directions to you; we have, however, come up with an awesome alternative. Once again, my good friends at coachdosmusic.com have created custom tracks that can be downloaded onto your MP3 player, thus allowing you to perform CHAOS drills by yourself. These drills are all made with custom work-to-rest ratios already built into each track. For example, a track may have 10 seconds of random direction changes followed by 30 seconds of rest. This track will continue until a total of 10 complete repetitions is completed. The result: a kick-butt workout that changes every time you put your headphones on. Visit coachdosmusic.com to download your free custom Coach Dos CHAOS tracks!

MORE TOOLS FOR OUR CARDIO STRENGTH TRAINING TOOLBOX

One of the things I enjoy doing when performing cardio strength workouts is training with my heart rate monitor on. Not only does the monitor tell me how things are going when compared to previous workouts, it can quantify my workouts by telling me the total cost (in calories) of that workout, my average heart rate, and, more importantly, my recovery rate for that particular session.

HEART RATE–BASED INTERVAL TRAINING

An alternative to timed rest periods during intervals is to actually let your body tell you when you are ready to perform the next repetition or work interval. As we train and get fit, our recovery can often be noted in how fast our heart rate comes down after a hard interval. While this is more pronounced in those of better-than-average fitness, it can often be difficult to control with beginners and even intermediate trainees. I'll give you an example.

Let's say we decide that someone with a resting heart rate of 80 beats per minute should get her heart rate all the way up to 160 beats per minute during a hard work interval. When using a heart rate–based rest interval, we would decide what would be a sufficient recovery heart rate. Many times we might just look for a 30-beat-per-minute drop or, in this case, say we want to see this trainee's heart rate get to 75 percent of her working heart rate. This would result in a target recovery heart rate of 130 if we used the 30-beat-per-minute drop or 112 if we used the 75 percent target number. At this point we would begin our next interval regardless of how long it took to get to this number. It could have been 20 seconds or it could have been a minute; it doesn't matter. As I already mentioned, with

Get creative with your anaerobic interval training. Sprints on a treadmill don't have to be followed by jogging. Jump off the treadmill and hit some body-weight, kettlebell, dumbbell, med ball, or barbell movements, then repeat.

Jim Smith, CSCS
Men's fitness expert
Co-founder of The Diesel Crew
dieselcrew.com

advanced trainees this recovery happens sooner; in fact, it often happens pretty darn close to the rest ratio numbers I have already mentioned in the previous chapters. The problem is that for a beginner or someone who is not as fit, it could take much, much longer for this heart rate to drop to our target number, sometimes upwards of 4 to 5 minutes. This now makes for some very long workout sessions. In these cases, you are better suited to use a timed interval regardless of the recovery heart rate.

Do I recommend using a heart rate monitor when doing your cardio strength training? Sure. Just keep in mind that many things like stress, sleep, fatigue, and so forth, can affect your heart rate any given day. Like I said, however, I do like to see how my recovery is going each session, how many calories I was able to burn in a specific training session, and my average heart rate for the entire session (a capability of many heart rate monitors).

I am a huge fan of pushing the sled for a number of reasons.

First, it fits right in with a number of athletic movements—from squats, to deadlifts, to Olympic lifts—that involve us transferring force from the lower body, through the core, to our upper body (and, in turn, the implement). So there is a fair amount of "general specificity" at work when you push a sled.

Second, it allows you to utilize a resistance training implement in a metabolic conditioning scenario without having to worry about technique breaking down with fatigue. When you get tired pushing the sled, you don't resort to bad (and potentially injurious) movement patterns to get the job done. Instead, you just hit a wall and the sled doesn't budge. With a lot of other complex resistance training movements, there is a big risk of injury secondary to poor form as fatigue sets in.

We'll push sleds with deliberate walking with long strides or more like a sprint. The distances are anywhere from 15 yards to 100 yards, and we'll vary the rest intervals. In many cases, we'll team up several athletes and have a set distance that they have to achieve as a team in a certain amount of time.

Eric Cressey, MS, CSCS
Author, Strength and Conditioning expert
ericcressey.com

CHANGING THE LANDSCAPE OF YOUR CARDIO STRENGTH TRAINING SESSIONS

I have already talked about getting out of the gym to do some sprint and agility training. In addition to this we can easily add intensity to many of our intervals by wearing a weighted vest, using medicine balls, doing our agility training in sand, and adding mini-bands into our jumps. In addition, you can perform timed intervals like Tabatas while using suspended rings (TRX), ropes, or push sleds, using a sledgehammer on a tire, or even flipping a strongman-style large tire for repetitions or time. See the next pages for a few of my favorite cardio strength workouts using some of these tools and accessories.

MORE INTERVAL EXERCISES				
EXERCISE	SLEDGEHAMMER STRIKING	TIRE FLIPS	PRO AGILITY IN SAND	ROPE BATTLE
Work:rest	15 seconds:15 seconds	30 seconds:30 seconds	5 seconds:25 seconds	30 seconds:30 seconds
Rounds	8	10	10	5
Total work time	4 minutes	10 minutes	5 minutes	5 minutes

SLEDGEHAMMER STRIKING

Using a heavy sledgehammer and a large tire to help absorb the shock, strike downward, trying to use your entire body to build momentum in each swing. Alternate your swings from your right shoulder to your left shoulder, making sure to let your arms extend fully and to let the rebound be completed before raising the sledgehammer overhead for your next strike.

TIRE FLIPS

Using an oversized tire and sitting in a deep squat with your fingers underneath or within the tire tread, deadlift the tire up, building momentum so that you are able to push the tire with your knee and finish by pushing the tire over.

PRO AGILITY IN SAND

This is the same pro agility drill diagrammed in the "Great Outdoors" chapter on page 201. The biggest difference is the sand surface that will make it much more difficult to run and accelerate off the stops.

ROPE BATTLE

Using a large manila or nylon rope (like the old climbing ropes in gym class), loop the rope around a sturdy base so that you have one end in each hand. Use a variety of patterns like alternating swings up and down, internal and external circles, and even jump squats with double arm swings. Use your entire body for these drills. You can emphasize more of your upper body by performing these drills on your knees as well.

MORE INTERVAL EXERCISES

EXERCISE	TRX OR RINGS— MOUNTAIN CLIMBERS & RING SQUAT JUMPS	MEDICINE BALL SLAMS	CHAOS SLIDES	SLED PUSHING
Work:rest	20 seconds:10 seconds	20 seconds:10 seconds	10 seconds:20 seconds	10 seconds:20 seconds
Rounds	8	8	10	10
Total work time	4 minutes	4 minutes	5 minutes	5 minutes

TRX OR SUSPENDED RING MOUNTAIN CLIMBERS

Holding the rings so that the straps are under your armpits, place your body in a 45-degree angle with your body straight and weight resting on your hands as the rings are set in your armpits. Forcefully perform mountain climbers, always keeping one foot off the floor and the opposite knee high into your stomach. Move as fast as possible in this drill.

TRX OR SUSPENDED RING SQUAT JUMPS

Stand holding the rings out in front of you with your arms extended. Move your feet slightly in front of you and lean back so that your weight is pulling on the rings. Squat deep and jump as high as possible as you simultaneously pull downward with your hands to help facilitate a greater jump. As you descend, offset your weight with your arms and sink back down into your next squat jump. You should almost be jumping in an arclike movement pattern due to the rings acting as an anchor.

MEDICINE BALL SLAMS

With your feet shoulder-width apart and holding a heavy medicine ball overhead, slam the ball down as hard as possible into the floor (slightly in front of your body), making sure to flex the torso and bring all of your core muscles into play on this movement. Catch the ball as it rebounds off the floor and move back into the fully extended start position before your next slam.

CHAOS SLIDES

Using the MP3 tracks, a partner acting as a rabbit, or someone yelling out direction changes, you will move as quickly as possible in a slide/shuffle pattern. Make sure to cover as much ground as possible and stop as quickly as possible on the direction changes. It should look as if you are sliding from side to side rather than bobbing up and down when you are shuffling.

SLED PUSHING

Using a sled dawg or other sled, keep your hips low and drive as hard and as fast as possible, making sure to fully extend your hips with every single push.

HIGH-POWERED NUTRITION

Once again I have the great pleasure to work with Mike Roussell as my nutrition expert on this book. As the author of the nutrition chapter in Men's Health Power Training, *Mike hit the performance nutrition scene with a bang! His nutrition principles and strategies have helped hundreds and hundreds of individuals reach their goals and Mike's future in this industry is as bright as it can be. This time around Mike focuses on high-powered nutrition, the type of nutrition to maximize your gains and performance in these often brutal cardio strength training workouts. I know you will enjoy and have great success following Mike's high-powered nutrition strategies.*

The cardio strength training methods presented in this book and in *Men's Health Power Training* by Coach Dos are some of the best you are going to find in regards to enhancing your metabolism, getting faster, getting stronger, and losing weight when time is a limiting factor. Because Coach Dos's training methods are so time efficient, it is important to do two things:

1. **Pour Maximum Effort into Each Session.** Cardio strength sessions are brutal—that is why they work. When you are done, your chest will be heaving and you might feel a little sick to your stomach. Toward the end of this chapter, we will go over some strategies that you can use to fight the nausea so you can train harder and get even better results.

2. **Properly Manage Your Nutrition the Other 23.5 Hours of the Day.** What you do nutritionally around your workout is very important, but how you manage your diet the rest of the day is even more important. In this chapter we will cover nutritional strategies that you can use around your workout and throughout the day to maximize the impact of your cardio strength training sessions.

OVERARCHING PRINCIPLES AND THE 6 PILLARS OF NUTRITION

If you look at the long-term nutrition studies where participants are asked to stick to a particular diet for longer than a 6-month period, you will see that adherence to the diet drops off significantly after 6 months. Why? People are busy (you're probably very busy and that is why the quick cardio strength training workouts are so appealing). Your diet needs to be able to function in the background of your life—fueling your activities and helping you mold the body you want while not getting in the way.

For this to happen, your diet needs to adhere to certain criteria—to be practical, simple, science based, and not require knowledge of vitamins or minerals. You need your diet to be practical and simple so that it is easy to follow even when your life gets busy. You need your diet to be based on real scientific research done on humans so that you know what you are doing works and aren't wasting your time with gimmicks, fads, and crazy protocols requiring cabbage, maple syrup, and only eating orange-colored foods the third Wednesday of each month. Finally, your diet should not require you to have any specialized knowledge of vitamins or minerals. This information is for the most part useless. You can lose weight, boost your health, and improve your fitness level without know-

ing anything about vitamins or minerals. All you need to know is a simple set of rules that will govern your food choices, and the rest will take care of itself. I call these rules The 6 Pillars of Nutrition.

I introduced The 6 Pillars of Nutrition in *Men's Health Power Training*, and it is warranted for them to be briefly mentioned again here as they serve as the foundation of your diet. For a more in-depth look at The 6 Pillars of Nutrition, see the nutrition chapter in *Power Training* or visit http://www.FreeNakedNutritionVideo.com.

THE 6 PILLARS OF NUTRITION

1. Eat Five to Six Times a Day.

2. Limit Your Consumption of Sugar and Processed Foods.

3. Eat Fruits and Vegetables Throughout the Day.

4. Drink More Water and Noncalorie-Containing Beverages.

5. Focus on Consuming Lean Protein Throughout the Day.

6. Save Starch Containing Foods Until after a Workout or for Breakfast.

Note: Starch-containing foods include rice, pasta, potatoes, oats, grains, and foods with added sugar (including sports drinks).

By following these six simple rules, you

will be able to maximize the effect of your cardio strength training workouts as you will be properly feeding your body throughout the day. While simple, The 6 Pillars of Nutrition are built on advanced nutritional strategies such as nutrient timing and strategic carbohydrate restriction.

NUTRITION FOR CARDIO STRENGTH TRAINING

Now let's move to a more specific look at how you can optimize your nutrition around your cardio strength training workouts to elicit their maximum benefit. The two areas that we will cover are enhancing performance and recovery and dealing with nausea.

ENHANCE PERFORMANCE AND RECOVERY

Many people use Coach Dos's cardio strength training to boost fat loss. If this is your goal, it is very important to realize that in order to achieve maximum fat loss you cannot be concerned with the number of calories from fat you burn during a particular training session. Instead, you need to focus on burning the greatest amount of total calories. This kind of intense exercise will force your body into burning calories (and fat) long after your workout is over as it tries to recover from your strength training cardio session.

Here are two strategies that you can employ to maximize your effort during your strength training cardio sessions:

1. **Drink Liquid Fast-Acting Protein and Carbohydrates before and after Your Training Session.** The one thing that I have seen that makes the greatest impact on my client's energy and performance in the gym is adding a liquid protein and carbohydrate drink before a training session. Timing a workout shake like this will prevent muscle breakdown, boost energy, and create the optimal hormonal environment for maximum recovery. Research has shown that protein- and carbohydrate-containing workout shakes increase muscle growth and do not hinder fat loss.

What to do: Make a shake that has a 2:1 ratio of carbs to protein. If you are doing just a strength training cardio session, you don't need a lot of calories in your shake; 10 to 15 grams of protein will suffice. If you are training more for strength and performance, then you can use a 3:1 ratio. If you are doing a cardio strength training session and a full workout, then you should use 25 to 30 grams of protein (adjust your carbohydrate intake according to the ratio you choose).

2. **Add a Performance Enhancer.** Beta-alanine is a dietary supplement that is perfectly suited to strength training cardio workouts. Beta-alanine is concentrated in your muscles and helps buffer the acidic

buildup caused by intense cardio strength training–type workouts. By adding a beta-alanine supplement to your plan of attack, you will be able to train longer and harder, and, as a result, you will burn more calories and see a greater improvement in your conditioning.

What to do: Take 4 to 6 grams total of beta-alanine spread out in 1- to 2-gram dosages throughout the day. It is necessary to spread out your intake of beta-alanine, as it has been reported in scientific studies and anecdotally to cause parenthesis (a "pins and needles" sensation on your skin) when taken in larger quantities. This side effect is completely harmless, but nevertheless annoying, so make sure to spread out your dosage over the course of the day.

DEALING WITH NAUSEA

Due to the intensity of cardio strength training workouts, one problem that you are almost guaranteed to run into is nausea. Here are some ways to help you keep your lunch from coming up and deal better with the nausea:

1. **Delay your workout.** For many people, having even a small workout shake in their stomach when they start a training session is a recipe for disaster (and vomit). If this is the case for you, simply increase the time between your preworkout shake and your cardio strength training workout.

2. **Use BCAAs instead.** Using branched chain amino acids (BCAAs) prior to a workout instead of a protein and carbohydrate workout shake is another good option if you have trouble working out shortly after having a shake. Mixing powdered (and flavored, as pure amino acids have a terrible taste) BCAAs in water and drinking that prior to your workout is much easier to stomach, as it feels more like you are just drinking water and the BCAAs do not sit in your stomach for very long.

3. **Control lactic acid.** Your feeling of nausea may be primarily driven by the increased levels of lactic acid that build up during strength training cardio sessions. Beta-alanine supplementation can help buffer lactic acid, which can also help with nausea.

4. **Eliminate stimulants.** Caffeine or caffeine plus yohimbe are commonly used as pre-workout stimulants. However, these may be counterproductive to cardio strength training sessions. If you are sensitive to stimulants, then the increased "energy boost" experienced from their use may contribute to your nausea. So if you are having trouble making it through a cardio strength training workout due to nausea, discontinue your preworkout stimulants.

5. **Give it time.** While this is not a nutritional intervention, the truth is it does not matter what you do, you are probably going to experience some level of nausea during your first couple weeks of cardio strength training workouts. As you continue to do these workouts, your conditioning will improve and the nausea will become more manageable.

YOUR HIGH-POWERED NUTRITION TOOLBOX

As we wrap up this chapter on using nutrition to maximize the effect of your strength training cardio session, it is important to walk away with a couple main points:

1. Regardless of all the workout nutrition tweaking you do, properly managing your nutrition outside of the gym and before your training sessions will have the greatest impact on your fat loss, strength, and performance.

2. You can increase the level of maximum effort your body is able to put into each workout by using a protein and carbohydrate shake prior to training and using a beta-alanine supplement throughout the day.

3. Due to the intensity of cardio strength training sessions, nausea may become an issue. You can reduce your feeling of nausea by waiting longer to work out after your preworkout shake, using a BCAA drink instead, controlling lactic acid through beta-alanine supplementation and better conditioning, and eliminating stimulants prior to your training session.

APPENDIX

COMPLEXES SAMPLE

INTERMEDIATE COMPLEXES WORKOUT LOGS			
INTERMEDIATE BARBELL COMPLEX	WEEKS 1–2	WEEKS 3–4	WEEKS 5–6
	3 X 6, 2 MINUTES REST	*3 X 7, 2 MINUTES REST*	*3 X 8, 90 SECONDS REST*
	WEIGHT USED	WEIGHT USED	WEIGHT USED
1. High pull	set #1—*55 lbs*	set #1—*65 lbs*	set #1—*65 lbs*
2. Drop lunge	set #2—*55 lbs*	set #2— *70 lbs*	set #2—*65 lbs*
3. Good morning	set #3—*60 lbs*	set #3—*70 lbs*	set #3—*65 lbs*
4. Ab rollout			

BEGINNER COMPLEXES

BEGINNER COMPLEXES WORKOUT LOGS			
BEGINNER BARBELL COMPLEX	**WEEKS 1–2**	**WEEKS 3–4**	**WEEKS 5–6**
	3 X 6, 2 MINUTES REST	*3 X 7, 2 MINUTES REST*	*3 X 8, 90 SECONDS REST*
	WEIGHT USED	**WEIGHT USED**	**WEIGHT USED**
1. Alternating lunge	set #1—	set #1—	set #1—
2. Good morning	set #2—	set #2—	set #2—
3. Push press	set #3—	set #3—	set #3—
BEGINNER DUMBBELL COMPLEX	**WEEKS 1–2**	**WEEKS 3–4**	**WEEKS 5–6**
	3 X 6, 2 MINUTES REST	*3 X 7, 2 MINUTES REST*	*3 X 8, 90 SECONDS REST*
	WEIGHT USED	**WEIGHT USED**	**WEIGHT USED**
1. Sumo deadlift	set #1—	set #1—	set #1—
2. Push press	set #2—	set #2—	set #2—
3. Bent-over alternating rows	set #3—	set #3—	set #3—
BEGINNER KETTLEBELL COMPLEX	**WEEKS 1–2**	**WEEKS 3–4**	**WEEKS 5–6**
	3 X 6, 2 MINUTES REST	*3 X 7, 2 MINUTES REST*	*3 X 8, 90 SECONDS REST*
	WEIGHT USED	**WEIGHT USED**	**WEIGHT USED**
1. Two-handed swing	set #1—	set #1—	set #1—
2. Bottoms-up sumo squat	set #2—	set #2—	set #2—
3. Push press	set #3—	set #3—	set #3—

BEGINNER COMPLEXES WORKOUT LOGS

BEGINNER BARBELL COMPLEX	WEEKS 7–8	WEEKS 9–10	WEEKS 11–12
	3 X 9, 90 SECONDS REST	*3 X 10, 75 SECONDS REST*	*3 X 10, 60 SECONDS REST*
	WEIGHT USED	**WEIGHT USED**	**WEIGHT USED**
1. Alternating lunge	set #1—	set #1—	set #1—
2. Good morning	set #2—	set #2—	set #2—
3. Push press	set #3—	set #3—	set #3—
BEGINNER DUMBBELL COMPLEX	WEEKS 7–8	WEEKS 9–10	WEEKS 11–12
	3 X 9, 90 SECONDS REST	*3 X 10, 75 SECONDS REST*	*3 X 10, 60 SECONDS REST*
	WEIGHT USED	**WEIGHT USED**	**WEIGHT USED**
1. Sumo deadlift	set #1—	set #1—	set #1—
2. Push press	set #2—	set #2—	set #2—
3. Bent-over alternating rows	set #3—	set #3—	set #3—
BEGINNER KETTLEBELL COMPLEX	WEEKS 7–8	WEEKS 9–10	WEEKS 11–12
	3 X 9, 90 SECONDS REST	*3 X 10, 75 SECONDS REST*	*3 X 10, 60 SECONDS REST*
	WEIGHT USED	**WEIGHT USED**	**WEIGHT USED**
1. Two-handed swing	set #1—	set #1—	set #1—
2. Bottoms-up sumo squat	set #2—	set #2—	set #2—
3. Push press	set #3—	set #3—	set #3—

INTERMEDIATE COMPLEXES

INTERMEDIATE COMPLEXES WORKOUT LOGS			
INTERMEDIATE BARBELL COMPLEX	**WEEKS 1–2**	**WEEKS 3–4**	**WEEKS 5–6**
	3 X 6, 2 MINUTES REST	*3 X 7, 2 MINUTES REST*	*3 X 8, 90 SECONDS REST*
	WEIGHT USED	**WEIGHT USED**	**WEIGHT USED**
1. High pull	set #1—	set #1—	set #1—
2. Drop lunge	set #2—	set #2—	set #2—
3. Good morning	set #3—	set #3—	set #3—
4. Barbell rollout			
INTERMEDIATE DUMBBELL COMPLEX	**WEEKS 1–2**	**WEEKS 3–4**	**WEEKS 5–6**
	3 X 6, 2 MINUTES REST	*3 X 7, 2 MINUTES REST*	*3 X 8, 90 SECONDS REST*
	WEIGHT USED	**WEIGHT USED**	**WEIGHT USED**
1. Curl-lunge-press hybrid	set #1—	set #1—	set #1—
2. Romanian deadlift	set #2—	set #2—	set #2—
3. Bent-over row	set #3—	set #3—	set #3—
4. Jump squat			
INTERMEDIATE KETTLEBELL COMPLEX	**WEEKS 1–2**	**WEEKS 3–4**	**WEEKS 5–6**
	3 X 6, 2 MINUTES REST	*3 X 7, 2 MINUTES REST*	*3 X 8, 90 SECONDS REST*
	WEIGHT USED	**WEIGHT USED**	**WEIGHT USED**
1. Alternating swing	set #1—	set #1—	set #1—
2. Clean and press (each arm)	set #2—	set #2—	set #2—
3. Windmill (each arm)	set #3—	set #3—	set #3—
4. Overhead squat (each arm)			

INTERMEDIATE COMPLEXES WORKOUT LOGS			
INTERMEDIATE BARBELL COMPLEX	**WEEKS 7–8**	**WEEKS 9–10**	**WEEKS 11–12**
	3 X 9, 90 SECONDS REST	*3 X 10, 75 SECONDS REST*	*3 X 10, 60 SECONDS REST*
	WEIGHT USED	**WEIGHT USED**	**WEIGHT USED**
1. High pull	set #1—	set #1—	set #1—
2. Drop lunge	set #2—	set #2—	set #2—
3. Good morning	set #3—	set #3—	set #3—
4. Ab rollout			
INTERMEDIATE DUMBBELL COMPLEX	**WEEKS 7–8**	**WEEKS 9–10**	**WEEKS 11–12**
	3 X 9, 90 SECONDS REST	*3 X 10, 75 SECONDS REST*	*3 X 10, 60 SECONDS REST*
	WEIGHT USED	**WEIGHT USED**	**WEIGHT USED**
1. Curl-lunge-press hybrid	set #1—	set #1—	set #1—
2. Romanian deadlift	set #2—	set #2—	set #2—
3. Bent-over row	set #3—	set #3—	set #3—
4. Jump squat			
INTERMEDIATE KETTLEBELL COMPLEX	**WEEKS 7–8**	**WEEKS 9–10**	**WEEKS 11–12**
	3 X 9, 90 SECONDS REST	*3 X 10, 75 SECONDS REST*	*3 X 10, 60 SECONDS REST*
	WEIGHT USED	**WEIGHT USED**	**WEIGHT USED**
1. Alternating swing	set #1—	set #1—	set #1—
2. Clean and press (each arm)	set #2—	set #2—	set #2—
3. Windmill (each arm)	set #3—	set #3—	set #3—
4. Overhead squat (each arm)			

ADVANCED COMPLEXES

ADVANCED COMPLEXES WORKOUT LOGS

ADVANCED BARBELL COMPLEX	WEEKS 1–2	WEEKS 3–4	WEEKS 5–6
	3 X 6, 2 minutes rest	*3 X 7, 2 minutes rest*	*3 X 8, 90 seconds rest*
	WEIGHT USED	WEIGHT USED	WEIGHT USED
1. Jump shrug	set #1—	set #1—	set #1—
2. Squat clean	set #2—	set #2—	set #2—
3. Push press	set #3—	set #3—	set #3—
4. Push press			
5. Hang snatch			
6. Overhead squat			
7. Bent-over row			
8. Romanian deadlift			
9. Plyometric pushups			
ADVANCED DUMBBELL COMPLEX	WEEKS 1–2	WEEKS 3–4	WEEKS 5–6
	3 X 6, 2 minutes rest	*3 X 7, 2 minutes rest*	*3 X 8, 90 seconds rest*
	WEIGHT USED	WEIGHT USED	WEIGHT USED
1. Hang snatch	set #1—	set #1—	set #1—
2. Squat and press hybrid	set #2—	set #2—	set #2—
3. Row and back extension hybrid	set #3—	set #3—	set #3—
4. Pushup and core row hybrid			
5. Weighted burpee			
ADVANCED KETTLEBELL COMPLEX	WEEKS 1–2	WEEKS 3–4	WEEKS 5–6
	3 X 6, 2 minutes rest	*3 X 7, 2 minutes rest*	*3 X 8, 90 seconds rest*
	WEIGHT USED	WEIGHT USED	WEIGHT USED
1. High pull	set #1—	set #1—	set #1—
2. Clean and push press hybrid	set #2—	set #2—	set #2—
3. Snatch	set #3—	set #3—	set #3—
4. Front squat			

ADVANCED COMPLEXES WORKOUT LOGS

ADVANCED BARBELL COMPLEX	WEEKS 7–8	WEEKS 9–10	WEEKS 11–12
	3 X 9, 90 SECONDS REST	*3 X 10, 75 SECONDS REST*	*3 X 10, 60 SECONDS REST*
	WEIGHT USED	WEIGHT USED	WEIGHT USED
1. Jump shrug	set #1—	set #1—	set #1—
2. Squat clean	set #2—	set #2—	set #2—
3. Push press	set #3—	set #3—	set #3—
4. Push press			
5. Hang snatch			
6. Overhead squat			
7. Bent-over row			
8. Romanian deadlift			
9. Plyometric pushups			
ADVANCED DUMBBELL COMPLEX	WEEKS 7–8	WEEKS 9–10	WEEKS 11–12
	3 X 9, 90 SECONDS REST	*3 X 10, 75 SECONDS REST*	*3 X 10, 60 SECONDS REST*
	WEIGHT USED	WEIGHT USED	WEIGHT USED
1. Hang snatch	set #1—	set #1—	set #1—
2. Squat and press hybrid	set #2—	set #2—	set #2—
3. Row and back extension hybrid	set #3—	set #3—	set #3—
4. Pushup and core row hybrid			
5. Weighted burpee			
ADVANCED KETTLEBELL COMPLEX	WEEKS 7–8	WEEKS 9–10	WEEKS 11–12
	3 X 9, 90 SECONDS REST	*3 X 10, 75 SECONDS REST*	*3 X 10, 60 SECONDS REST*
	WEIGHT USED	WEIGHT USED	WEIGHT USED
1. High pull	set #1—	set #1—	set #1—
2. Clean and push press hybrid	set #2—	set #2—	set #2—
3. Snatch	set #3—	set #3—	set #3—
4. Front squat			

DENSITY SAMPLE

DENSITY TRAINING WORKOUT LOGS				
DENSITY CIRCUIT MENU	EXERCISES	WEIGHT USED	TIME OF CIRCUIT	SETS COMPLETED
Date: 4/24/09			20 minutes	19 sets
Explosive	Bulgarian split jumps	20-lb vest		
Knee/Hip dominant	DB 1-leg RDL	85 lbs		
Upper body push	DB bench press	90 lbs		
Upper body pull	Chinups	20-lb vest		
Core	Barbell situp	70 lbs		

DENSITY WORKOUT LOGS

DENSITY TRAINING WORKOUT LOGS				
DENSITY CIRCUIT MENU	**EXERCISES**	**WEIGHT USED**	**TIME OF CIRCUIT**	**SETS COMPLETED**
Date:				
Explosive				
Knee/Hip dominant				
Upper body push				
Upper body pull				
Core				
DENSITY CIRCUIT MENU	**EXERCISES**	**WEIGHT USED**	**TIME OF CIRCUIT**	**SETS COMPLETED**
Date:				
Explosive				
Knee/Hip dominant				
Upper body push				
Upper body pull				
Core				
DENSITY CIRCUIT MENU	**EXERCISES**	**WEIGHT USED**	**TIME OF CIRCUIT**	**SETS COMPLETED**
Date:				
Explosive				
Knee/Hip dominant				
Upper body push				
Upper body pull				
Core				

DENSITY CIRCUIT MENU	EXERCISES	WEIGHT USED	TIME OF CIRCUIT	SETS COMPLETED
Date:				
Explosive				
Knee/Hip dominant				
Upper body push				
Upper body pull				
Core				
DENSITY CIRCUIT MENU	EXERCISES	WEIGHT USED	TIME OF CIRCUIT	SETS COMPLETED
Date:				
Explosive				
Knee/Hip dominant				
Upper body push				
Upper body pull				
Core				

INDEX

Boldface page references indicate photographs. <u>Underscored</u> references indicate boxed text.

A

Ab rollout, 66, **66**, 157, **157**
Aerobic fitness, 7
Aerobic intervals, 201–2
Afterburn, 1, 47
Agility training
    CHAOS, 205–6, <u>206</u>
    description of, 203–4
    five and back/10 and backs, **203**, 204
    pro agility (5/10/5 drill), 204, **204**
    sample workout, <u>205</u>
    warmup for, 15
AirDyne, use in Tabatas, <u>116</u>
Alternating lunge
    barbell, 54, **54**
    body-weight, 28, **28**
Alternating swing, 71, **71**
Anaerobic threshold, 202
Atlas lunge, 37, **37**

B

Back squat, 48, **48**, 127, **127**
Barbell complex
    advanced, 75–81, **75–81**
        hang snatch, 78, **78**
        jump shrug, 75, **75**
        overhead squat, 79, **79**
        plyometric pushups, 81, **81**
        push press, 77, **77**
        Romanian deadlift, 80, **80**
        squat clean, 76, **76**
    beginner, 54–56, **54–56**
        alternating lunge, 54, **54**
        good morning, 55, **55**
        push press, 56, **56**
    intermediate, 63–66, **63–66**
        ab rollout, 66, **66**, 226, 229, 230
        drop lunge, 64, **64**
        good morning, 65, **65**
        high pull, 63, **63**
    starter, 48–49, **48–49**
        back squat, 48, **48**
        behind-the-neck push press, 49, **49**
    warmup, 16–21, **16–21**
        bent-over row, 20, **20**
        front squat, 19, **19**
        hang jump shrug, 16, **16**
        hang power clean, 17, **17**
        push press, 18, **18**
        Romanian deadlift, 21, **21**

Barbell situps, 153, **153**
BCAAs, 222, 223
Behind-the-neck push press, 49, **49**
Bench press, 133, **133**
Bent-over alternating row, 25, **25**, 59, **59**
Bent-over row
    barbell, 20, **20**, 148, **148**
    dumbbell, 69, **69**
Beta-alanine, 221–22, 223
Body-weight complex
    complex #1, 93–97, **93–97**
        burpees, 96, **96**
        mountain climbers, 97, **97**
        plyometric pushups, 95, **95**
        split jumps, 94, **94**
        squats, 93, **93**
    complex #2, 98–101, **98–101**
        burpee and pullup hybrid, 98, **98**
        leg raises, 101, **101**
        plyometric pushups, 100, **100**
        squat jump, 99, **99**
    warmup, 28–33, **28–33**
        alternating lunges, 28, **28**
        burpees, 30, **30**
        mountain climbers, 32, **32**
        pushups, 31, **31**
        side squats, 33, **33**
        squat jumps, 29, **29**
Bottoms-up sumo squat, 61, **61**
Branched chain amino acids (BCAAs), 222, 223
Bulgarian split jump, 125, **125**
Bulgarian split squat, 129, **129**
Burpee and pullup hybrid, 98, **98**
Burpees, 30, **30**, 96, **96**

C

Cable complex, 90–92, **90–92**
    split squat and press hybrid, 92, **92**
    squat and row hybrid, 90, **90**
    woodchop, 91, **91**
Cable face pulls, 149, **149**
Cable push-pull anti-rotation, 156, **156**
Cable woodchop (high to low), 155, **155**
Cable woodchop (low to high), 154, **154**
Caffeine, 222
Calisthenics, 11
Carbohydrates, in workout shake, 221, 223
Cardio strength training
    benefits of, 2, 7
    description of, 1–3

expectations from, 3
modes, 9–12
  complexes, 9
  density training, 9–10
  heart rate-based training, 11–12
  on and off circuits, 10
  old school training, 11
  traditional repetition sets, 10–11
science behind, 5–8
Carioca stepover, 36, **36**
CHAOS agility training, 205–6, <u>206</u>
CHAOS slides, 217, <u>217</u>
Chinups, 143, **143**
Clean and press, 72, **72**
Clean and push press hybrid, 87, **87**
Complexes
  advanced
    barbell, 75–81, **75–81**
    description of, 43, <u>43</u>
    dumbbell, 82–85, **82–85**
    kettlebell, 86–89, **86–89**
    workout logs, <u>231–32</u>
  beginner
    barbell, 54–56, **54–56**
    description of, 43, <u>43</u>
    dumbbell, 57–59, **57–59**
    kettlebell, 60–62, **60–62**
    workout logs, <u>227–28</u>
  body weight #1, 93–97, **93–97**
  body weight #2, 98–101, **98–101**
  cable, 90–92, **90–92**
  components of, 42
  description of, 9, 13
  intermediate
    barbell, 63–66, **63–66**
    description of, 44, <u>44</u>
    dumbbell, 67–70, **67–70**
    kettlebell, 71–74, **71–74**
    workout logs, <u>229–30</u>
  as king of cardio strength training, 41
  load choice, 43
  origin of concept, 42, <u>42</u>
  place in training schedule, 46–47
  progressions, 43, 45, <u>45</u>
  recovery, 46
  repetition number, choosing, 42–43
  rest periods, 45, 45, 46
  rules for performing, 42
  starter
    barbell, 48–49, **48–49**
    description of, 43, <u>43</u>
    dumbbell, 50–51, **50–51**
    kettlebell, 52–53, **52–53**
  suspended rings, 102–5, **102–5**
  tools for performing, <u>46</u>, 47, <u>89</u>
  warmup
    barbell, 16–21

    body-weight, 28–33
    dumbbell, 22–27
  workout logs
    advanced, <u>231–32</u>
    beginner, <u>227–28</u>
    intermediate, <u>229–30</u>
    sample, <u>226</u>
Cooldown, 15
Core exercises, 151–58, **151–58**
  ab rollout, 157, **157**
  barbell situps, 153, **153**
  cable push-pull anti-rotation, 156, **156**
  cable woodchop (high to low), 155, **155**
  cable woodchop (low to high), 154, **154**
  standing barbell anti-rotation, 152, **152**
  superman pushups, 151, **151**
  windmills, 158, **158**
Core row, 27, **27**
Countdowns, 114, <u>114</u>
Curl-lunge-press hybrid, 67, **67**

D
Deadlift
  Romanian
    barbell, 21, **21**, 80, **80**, 159, **159**
    dumbbell, 68, **68**
    dumbbell one-leg, 162, **162**
  sumo, 57, **57**
Density training
  circuit setup, 107–8
  core exercises, 151–58, **151–58**
    ab rollout, 157, **157**
    barbell situps, 153, **153**
    cable push-pull anti-rotation, 156, **156**
    cable woodchop (high to low), 155, **155**
    cable woodchop (low to high), 154, **154**
    standing barbell anti-rotation, 152, **152**
    superman pushups, 151, **151**
    windmills, 158, **158**
  description of, 9–10
  Escalating Density Training (EDT), 108
  exercise menu, <u>108</u>, <u>109</u>, 109–10, <u>110</u>
  explosive exercises, 117–25, **117–25**
    Bulgarian split jump, 125, **125**
    dumbbell burpees, 124, **124**
    hang clean, 122, **122**
    hang snatch, 123, **123**
    jump shrug, 121, **121**
    jump squat, 117, **117**
    kettlebell alternating swing, 119, **119**
    kettlebell snatch, 120, **120**
    seated pause box jump, 118, **118**
  favorite combinations, 110, <u>111–13</u>
  hip-dominant exercises, 159–65, **159–65**
    dumbbell one-leg Romanian deadlift, 162, **162**
    good morning, 160, **160**
    one-leg back extension, 161, **161**

Density training (cont.)
  hip-dominant exercises (cont.)
    Romanian deadlift, 159, **159**
    seated good morning, 163, **163**
    stability ball leg curl, 164, **164**
    val slide leg curl, 165, **165**
  knee-dominant exercises, 126–32, **126–32**
    back squat, 127, **127**
    Bulgarian split squat, 129, **129**
    drop lunge, 130, **130**
    front squat, 126, **126**
    overhead squat, 128, **128**
    single-leg squat, 131, **131**
    split squat, 132, **132**
  rules for, 108
  upper body pull exercises, 142–50, **142–50**
    bent-over row, 148, **148**
    cable face pulls, 149, **149**
    chinups, 143, **143**
    horizontal pullups, 145, **145**
    one-arm dumbbell plank row, 150, **150**
    one-arm horizontal pullup, 147, **147**
    pullups, 142, **142**
    side-to-side pullups, 144, **144**
    suspended rows, 146, **146**
  upper body push exercises, 133–41, **133–41**
    bench press, 133, **133**
    dips, 140, **140**
    dumbbell alternating bench press, 135, **135**
    dumbbell half bench press, 136, **136**
    dumbbell push press, 139, **139**
    incline press, 134, **134**
    push jerk, 138, **138**
    push press, 137, **137**
    suspended pushup, 141, **141**
Dietary supplement, 221–22, 223
Dips, 140, **140**
Drop lunge, 64, **64**, 130, **130**
Dumbbell alternating bench press, 135, **135**
Dumbbell burpees, 124, **124**
Dumbbell complex
  advanced, 82–85, **82–85**
    hang snatch, 82, **82**
    pushup and core row hybrid, 84, **84**
    squat and press hybrid, 83, **83**
    weighted burpee, 85, **85**
  beginner, 57–59, **57–59**
    bent-over alternating row, 59, **59**
    push press, 58, 58
    sumo deadlift, 57, **57**
  intermediate, 67–70, **67–70**
    bent-over row, 69, **69**
    curl-lunge-press hybrid, 67, **67**
    jump squat, 70, **70**
    Romanian deadlift, 68, **68**
  starter, 50–51, **50–51**
    front squat, 50, **50**
    push press, 51, **51**

    warmup, 22–27, **22–27**
      bent-over alternating row, 25, **25**
      core row, 27, **27**
      hang snatch, 23, **23**
      high pull, 22, **22**
      pushup, 26, **26**
      squat and press, 24, **24**
Dumbbell half bench press, 136, **136**
Dumbbell one-leg Romanian deadlift, 162, **162**
Dumbbell push press, 139, **139**
Dumbbell sumo squat + curl and press, 189, **189**
Dynamic warmups, 34–40, **34–40**
  atlas lunge (10 yards), 37, **37**
  carioca stepover (15 yards), 36, **36**
  knee skips, 34, **34**
  lateral 180-degree squats (10 yards), 38, **38**
  leg swings, 35, **35**
  repetitions and distance, 14
  spiderman lunge (10 yards), 39, **39**
  three-quater speed accelerations (20 yards),
    40, **40**

E
Escalating Density Training (EDT), 108
Excess Postexercise Oxygen Consumption (EPOC),
  47
Exercises
  ab rollout, 66, **66**, 157, **157**
  alternating lunge
    barbell, 54, **54**
    body-weight, 28, **28**
  alternating swing, 71, **71**
  atlas lunge, 37, **37**
  back squat, 48, **48**, 127, **127**
  barbell situps, 153, **153**
  behind-the-neck push press, 49, **49**
  bench press, 133, **133**
  bent-over alternating row, 25, **25**, 59, **59**
  bent-over row
    barbell, 20, **20**, 148, **148**
    dumbbell, 69, **69**
  bottoms-up sumo squat, 61, **61**
  Bulgarian split jump, 125, **125**
  Bulgarian split squat, 129, **129**
  burpee and pullup hybrid, 98, **98**
  burpees, 30, **30**, 96, **96**
  cable face pulls, 149, **149**
  cable push-pull anti-rotation, 156, **156**
  cable woodchop (high to low), 155, **155**
  cable woodchop (low to high), 154, **154**
  carioca stepover, 36, **36**
  chaos slides, 217, **217**
  chinups, 143, **143**
  clean and press, 72, **72**
  clean and push press hybrid, 87, **87**
  core row, 27, **27**
  curl-lunge-press hybrid, 67, **67**
  dips, 140, **140**

drop lunge, 64, **64**, 130, **130**
dumbbell alternating bench press, 135, **135**
dumbbell burpees, 124, **124**
dumbbell half bench press, 136, **136**
dumbbell push press, 139, **139**
five and back/10 and backs, **203**, 204
front squat
    barbell, 19, **19**, 126, **126**
    dumbbell, 50, **50**
    kettlebell, 89, **89**
good morning, 55, **55**, 65, **65**, 160, **160**
hang clean, 122, **122**
hang jump shrug, 16, **16**
hang power clean, 17, **17**
hang snatch
    barbell, 78, **78**, 123, **123**
    dumbbell, 23, **23**, 82, **82**
heavy bag punching/kicking, 195, **195**
high pull
    barbell, 63, **63**
    dumbbell, 22, **22**
    kettlebell, 86, **86**
horizontal pullups, 145, **145**
horizontal rows, 102, **102**
ice skaters, 105, **105**
incline press, 134, **134**
jump rope, 194, **194**
jump shrug
    barbell, 75, **75**
    kettlebell, 121, **121**
jump squat, 117, **117**
    dumbbell, 70, **70**
    on suspended rings, 103, **103**
kettlebell alternating swing, 119, **119**, 176, **176**
kettlebell front squat (one sided), 170, **170**
kettlebell snatch, 120, **120**
kettlebell sumo jump squat, 171, **171**
kettlebell swing, 174, **174**
knee skips, 34, **34**
lateral 180-degree squats, 38, **38**
leg raises, 101, **101**
leg swings, 35, **35**
medicine ball burpee, 186, **186**
medicine ball mountain climbers, 199, **199**
medicine ball overhead squat, 185, **185**
medicine ball plyo pushups, 197, **197**
medicine ball pushup, 183, **183**
medicine ball slams, 216, **216**
medicine ball split jump, 182, **182**
medicine ball split squat jumps, 200, **200**
medicine ball squat jumps, 198, **198**
medicine ball straight leg situp, 184, **184**
mountain climbers, 32, **32**, 97, **97**
    with medicine ball, 199, **199**
one-arm dumbbell plank row, 150, **150**
one-arm horizontal pullup, 147, **147**
one-leg back extension, 161, **161**

overhead squat
    barbell, 79, **79**, 128, **128**
    kettlebell, 74, **74**
plank walkup, 167, **167**
plank with weight transfer, 169, **169**
plyometric pushups, 81, **81**, 95, **95**, 100, **100**
    in countdowns, 114, 114
    with medicine ball, 197, **197**
pro agility (5/10/5 drill), 204, **204**
pro agility in sand, 212, **212**
pullups, 142, **142**
push jerk, 138, **138**
push press
    barbell, 18, **18**, 56, **56**, 77, **77**, 137, **137**
    dumbbell, 51, **51**, 58, **58**, 58
    kettlebell, 62, **62**
pushup and core row hybrid, 84, **84**
pushups
    on dumbbells, 26, **26**, 84, **84**
    medicine ball, 183, **183**
    medicine ball plyo pushups, 197, **197**
    plyometric, 81, **81**, 95, **95**, 100, **100**, 114, 114
    standard, 31, **31**
    superman, 151, **151**
    on suspended rings, 104, **104**, 141, **141**
    TRX atomic, 178, **178**
    val slide atomic, 173, **173**
reverse lunge, 166, **166**
Romanian deadlift
    barbell, 21, **21**, 80, **80**, 159, **159**
    dumbbell, 68, **68**
    dumbbell one-leg, 162, **162**
rope battle, 213, **213**
seated good morning, 163, **163**
seated pause box jump, 118, **118**
side squats, 33, **33**
side-to-side pullups, 144, **144**
single-leg squat, 131, **131**
sledgehammer striking, 210, **210**
sled pushing, 208, 218, **218**
snatch, 88, **88**
speed jumps, 196, **196**
spiderman lunge, 39, **39**
split jumps, 94, **94**
split squat, 132, **132**
split squat and press hybrid, 92, **92**
split squat jump, 168, **168**
    with medicine ball, 200, **200**
squat, 93, **93**
squat and press, 24, **24**
squat and press hybrid, 83, **83**
squat and row hybrid, 90, **90**
squat clean, 76, **76**
squat jump, 29, **29**, 99, **99**
    in countdowns, 114, 114
    with medicine ball, 198, **198**
stability ball leg curl, 164, **164**
standing barbell anti-rotation, 152, **152**

Exercises (cont.)
  sumo deadlift, 57, **57**
  sumo squat, 53, **53**
  sumo squat + curl and press, 189, **189**
  superman pushups, 151, **151**
  suspended pushup, 141, **141**
  suspended rows, 146, **146**
  three-quater speed accelerations, 40, **40**
  tire flips, 211, **211**
  TRX 180 degree jumps, 179, **179**
  TRX atomic pushup, 178, **178**
  TRX rows, 180, **180**
  TRX superman, 181, **181**
  TRX/suspended ring jump squats, 215, **215**
  TRX/suspended ring mountain climbers, 214, **214**
  two-handed swing, 52, **52**, 60, **60**, 187, **187**, 188,
    188
  val slide ab slide, 175, **175**
  val slide atomic pushup, 173, **173**
  val slide leg curl, 165, **165**
  val slide sled push, 177, **177**
  weighted burpee, 85, **85**
  windmills, 73, **73**, 158, **158**
  woodchop, 91, **91**
Explosive exercises, 117–25, **117–25**
  Bulgarian split jump, 125, **125**
  dumbbell burpees, 124, **124**
  hang clean, 122, **122**
  hang snatch, 123, **123**
  jump shrug, 121, **121**
  jump squat, 117, **117**
  kettlebell alternating swing, 119, **119**
  kettlebell snatch, 120, **120**
  seated pause box jump, 118, **118**

F
Fat-burning exercise, 1–2
Fat loss, interval training and, 2, 7
Five and back/10 and backs, **203**, 204
5/10/5 drill, 204, **204**
Front squat, 126, **126**
  barbell, 19, **19**, 126, **126**
  dumbbell, 50, **50**
  kettlebell, 89, **89**
Functional capacity, 3

G
Good morning, 55, **55**, 65, **65**, 160, **160**
Greasing the knees, 14

H
Hang clean, 122, **122**
Hang jump shrug, 16, **16**
Hang power clean, 17, **17**
Hang snatch, 123, **123**
  barbell, 78, **78**, 123, **123**
  dumbbell, 23, **23**, 82, **82**

Heart rate
  lowering after training session, 15
  as measure of intensity, 3
Heart rate-based interval training, 11–12, 207–8
Heart rate monitor, 11–12, 207–8
Heavy bag punching/kicking, 195, **195**
High-intensity interval training. *See also* Intervals
  benefits of
    aerobic fitness, 2, 7
    fat loss, 2, 7
    steady-state aerobics compared, 6–7
    time required for, 6–7
High pull
  barbell, 63, **63**
  dumbbell, 22, **22**
  kettlebell, 86, **86**
Hip-dominant exercises, 159–65, **159–65**
  dumbbell one-leg Romanian deadlift, 162, **162**
  good morning, 160, **160**
  one-leg back extension, 161, **161**
  Romanian deadlift, 159, **159**
  seated good morning, 163, **163**
  stability ball leg curl, 164, **164**
  val slide leg curl, 165, **165**
Horizontal pullups, 145, **145**
Horizontal rows, 102, **102**

I
Ice skaters, 105, **105**
Incline press, 134, **134**
Intensity
  heart rate as measure of, 3
  of intervals, 10
Intervals
  aerobic, 201–2
  agility training, **203**, 203–6, **204**, 205
  anaerobic, 202, 208
  benefits of, 2
  breaking into short bouts, 10
  exercises
    chaos slides, 217, **217**
    medicine ball slams, 216, **216**
    pro agility in sand, 212, **212**
    rope battle, 213, **213**
    sledgehammer striking, 210, **210**
    sled pushing, 208, 218, **218**
    tire flips, 211, **211**
    TRX/suspended ring jump squats, 215, **215**
    TRX/suspended ring mountain climbers, 214,
      214
  heart rate-based, 11–12, 207–8
  intensity, 10
  sprint, 201–3, 202, 203
  using 30 seconds work: 30-second rest intervals, 10–11,
    111, 111–12, 170, 170–71, **170–71**
    kettlebell front squat (one sided), 170, **170**
    kettlebell sumo jump squat, 171, **171**

using 30 seconds work: 60-second rest intervals, 110, 111, 166, 166–69, **166–69**
    plank walkup, 167, **167**
    plank with weight transfer, 169, **169**
    reverse lunge, 166, **166**
    split squat jump, 168, **168**
using 30 seconds work: 90-second rest intervals, 112–13, 113
using 40 seconds work: 20-second rest intervals, 112, 112, 172, 173–84, **173–84**, 173–86, **173–86**
    kettlebell alternating swing, 176, **176**
    kettlebell swing, 174, **174**
    medicine ball burpee, 186, **186**
    medicine ball overhead squat, 185, **185**
    medicine ball pushup, 183, **183**
    medicine ball split jump, 182, **182**
    medicine ball straight leg situp, 184, **184**
    TRX 180 degree jumps, 179, **179**
    TRX atomic pushup, 178, **178**
    TRX rows, 180, **180**
    TRX superman, 181, **181**
    val slide ab slide, 175, **175**
    val slide atomic pushup, 173, **173**
    val slide sled push, 177, **177**
    workout #1, 173–77, **173–77**
    workout #2, 178–81, **178–81**
    workout #3, 181–84, **181–84**

J

Jogging, for cooldown, 15
Jump rope, 194, **194**
Jump shrug, 121, **121**
    barbell, 75, **75**
    kettlebell, 121, **121**
Jump squats, 117, **117**
    dumbbell, 70, **70**
    on suspended rings, 103, **103**
    TRX/suspended ring, 215, **215**

K

Kettlebell alternating swing, 119, **119**, 176, **176**
Kettlebell complex
    advanced, 86–89, **86–89**
        clean and push press hybrid, 87, **87**
        front squat, 89, **89**
        high pull, 86, **86**
        snatch, 88, **88**
    beginner, 60–62, **60–62**
        bottoms-up sumo squat, 61, **61**
        push press, 62, **62**
        two-handed swing, 60, **60**
    benefits of, 2
    intermediate, 71–74, **71–74**
        alternating swing, 71, **71**
        clean and press, 72, **72**
        overhead squat, 74, **74**
        windmill, 73, **73**

    starter, 52–53, **52–53**
        sumo squat, 53, **53**
        two-handed swing, 52, **52**
Kettlebell front squat (one sided), 170, **170**
Kettlebells, benefits of, 44
Kettlebell snatch, 120, **120**
Kettlebell sumo jump squat, 171, **171**
Kettlebell swing, 174, **174**
Kettlebell two-handed swing, 187, **187**
Kicking (heavy bag), 195, **195**
Knee-dominant exercises, 126–32, **126–32**
    back squat, 127, **127**
    Bulgarian split squat, 129, **129**
    drop lunge, 130, **130**
    front squat, 126, **126**
    overhead squat, 128, **128**
    single-leg squat, 131, **131**
    split squat, 132, **132**
Knees, greasing, 14
Knee skips, 34, **34**

L

Lactic acid, controlling, 222, 223
Lateral 180-degree squats, 38, **38**
Leg raises, 101, **101**
Leg swings, 35, **35**
Logs. *See* Workout logs
Lunges
    alternating
        barbell, 54, **54**
        body-weight, 28, **28**
    atlas, 37, **37**
    curl-lunge-press hybrid, 67, **67**
    drop, 64, **64**, 130, **130**
    reverse, 166, **166**
    spiderman, 39, **39**

M

Medicine ball burpee, 186, **186**
Medicine ball mountain climbers, 199, **199**
Medicine ball overhead squat, 185, **185**
Medicine ball plyo pushups, 197, **197**
Medicine ball pushup, 183, **183**
Medicine ball slams, 216, **216**
Medicine ball split jump, 182, **182**
Medicine ball split squat jumps, 200, **200**
Medicine ball squat jumps, 198, **198**
Medicine ball straight leg situp, 184, **184**
Metabolic rate, postexercise, 6
Metabolic training, 3
Mountain climbers, 32, **32**, 97, **97**
    with medicine ball, 199, **199**
    TRX/suspended ring, 214, **214**

N

Nausea, dealing with, 222–23
Negative rest intervals, 115

Nutrition, 219–23
    dealing with nausea, 222–23
    to enhance performance and recovery, 221–22
    6 pillars of, 220–21

O

On and off circuits, 10
One-arm dumbbell plank row, 150, **150**
One-arm horizontal pullup, 147, **147**
One-leg back extension, 161, **161**
Outdoor training
    agility training, 203–6
    sprint training, 201–3
Overhead squat
    barbell, 79, **79**, 128, **128**
    kettlebell, 74, **74**
    medicine ball, 185, **185**
Overload principle, 3

P

Plank walkup, 167, **167**
Plank with weight transfer, 169, **169**
Plyometric pushups, 81, **81**, 95, **95**, 100, **100**
    in countdowns, 114, 114
    with medicine ball, 197, **197**
Pre-fatiguing, 3
Pro agility drill, 204, **204**
    in sand, 212, **212**
Progressive overload, complexes for, 45, 45
Protein, in workout shake, 221, 223
Pullups, 142, **142**
Punching (heavy bag), 195, **195**
Push jerk, 138, **138**
Push press
    barbell, 18, **18**, 56, **56**, 77, **77**, 137, **137**
    dumbbell, 51, **51**, 58, 58
    kettlebell, 62, **62**
Push sled, 208, 218, **218**
Pushup and core row hybrid, 84, **84**
Pushups
    core row hybrid, 84, **84**
    with dumbbells, 26, **26**, 84, **84**
    medicine ball, 183, **183**
    medicine ball plyo pushups, 197, **197**
    plyometric, 81, **81**, 95, **95**, 100, **100**, 114, 114
    standard, 31, **31**
    superman, 151, **151**
    on suspended rings, 104, **104**, 141, **141**
    TRX atomic, 178, **178**
    val slide atomic, 173, **173**

R

Recovery
    in complex sets, 46
    nutrition and, 221–22
Repetition counting circuits
    20/10s, 115
    24s, 113, 113
    countdowns, 114, 114

Rest intervals
    in complex sets, 45, 45, 46
    in density training workout, 109
    negative, 115
    in Tabatas, 115
    in timed sets, 110–14
Reverse lunge, 166, **166**
Romanian deadlift
    barbell, 21, **21**, 80, **80**, 159, **159**
    dumbbell, 68, **68**
    dumbbell one-leg, 162, **162**
Rope battle, 213, **213**
Runners, body fat of, 5

S

Sand, pro agility drill in, 212, **212**
Seated good morning, 163, **163**
Seated pause box jump, 118, **118**
Shake, 221, 222, 223
Side squats, 33, **33**
Side-to-side pullups, 144, **144**
Single-leg squat, 131, **131**
6 pillars of nutrition, 220–21
Sledgehammer striking, 210, **210**
Sled pushing, 208, 218, **218**
Snatch, 88, **88**
Speed jumps, 196, **196**
Spiderman lunge, 39, **39**
Split jumps, 94, **94**
Split squat, 132, **132**
    Bulgarian, 129, **129**
Split squat and press hybrid, 92, **92**
Split squat jump, 168, **168**
    with medicine ball, 200, **200**
Sprint training
    aerobic *versus* anaerobic, 201–2
    agility drills, 203, 203–6, **204**, 205
    distances, 202, 202, 203
    sample workouts, 203
    warmup for, 15
    work-to-rest ratios, 202, 202–3
Squat and press, 24, **24**
Squat and press hybrid, 83, **83**
Squat and row hybrid, 90, **90**
Squat clean, 76, **76**
Squat jump, 29, **29**, 99, **99**
    in countdowns, 114, 114
    with medicine ball, 198, **198**
Squats, 93, **93**
    back, 48, **48**, 127, **127**
    front squat
        barbell, 19, **19**, 126, **126**
        dumbbell, 50, **50**
        kettlebell, 89, **89**, 170, **170**
    jump squat, 117, **117**
        dumbbell, 70, **70**
        on suspended rings, 103, **103**
        TRX/suspended ring, 215, **215**

kettlebell sumo jump squat, 171, **171**
lateral 180-degree, 38, **38**
overhead squat
    barbell, 79, **79**, 128, **128**
    kettlebell, 74, **74**
    medicine ball, 185, **185**
side, 33, **33**
single-leg, 131, **131**
split squat, 132, **132**
    Bulgarian, 129, **129**
split squat and press hybrid, 92, **92**
split squat jump, 168, **168**
    with medicine ball, 200, **200**
squat and press, 24, **24**
squat and press hybrid, 83, **83**
squat and row hybrid, 90, **90**
squat clean, 76, **76**
squat jump, 29, **29**, 99, **99**
    in countdowns, 114, 114
    with medicine ball, 198, **198**
sumo squat, 53, **53**
    bottoms-up, 61, **61**
sumo squat + curl and press, 189, **189**
Stability ball leg curl, 164, **164**
Standing barbell anti-rotation, 152, **152**
Stimulants, eliminating preworkout, 222, 223
Sumo deadlift, 57, **57**
Sumo squat, 53, **53**
    bottoms-up, 61, **61**
Sumo squat + curl and press, 189, **189**
Superman pushups, 151, **151**
Supplement, dietary, 221–22, 223
Suspended pushup, 141, **141**
Suspended rings complex, 102–5, **102–5**
    horizontal rows, 102, **102**
    ice skaters, 105, **105**
    jump squats, 103, **103**
    pushups, 104, **104**
Suspended rows, 146, **146**

T

Tabatas
    aerobic fitness from, 7
    AirDyne use in, 116
    description of, 191–92
    exercises
        heavy bag punching/kicking, 195, **195**
        jump rope, 194, **194**
        medicine ball mountain climbers, 199, **199**
        medicine ball plyo pushups, 197, **197**
        medicine ball split squat jumps, 200, **200**
        medicine ball squat jumps, 198, **198**
        speed jumps, 196, **196**
    external load use in, 115, 115–16
    favorite exercise movements, 192, 192–93
    favorite exercise sequences, 193, 193
    modifications
        10-second work: 20-second rest interval, 192

        15-second work: 15-second rest interval, 192
        20-second work: 10-second rest interval, 192
    negative rest intervals, 115
    spin-offs of, 191
Three-quater speed accelerations, 40, **40**
Timed sets. *See also* Density training
    barbell Tabata exercise
        two-handed swing, 188, **188**
    benefits of, 108, 109
    core exercises, 151–58, **151–58**
        ab rollout, 157, **157**
        barbell situps, 153, **153**
        cable push-pull anti-rotation, 156, **156**
        cable woodchop (high to low), 155, **155**
        cable woodchop (low to high), 154, **154**
        standing barbell anti-rotation, 152, **152**
        superman pushups, 151, **151**
        windmills, 158, **158**
    dumbbell Tabata exercise
        sumo squat + curl and press, 189, **189**
    explosive exercises, 117–25, **117–25**
        Bulgarian split jump, 125, **125**
        dumbbell burpees, 124, **124**
        hang clean, 122, **122**
        hang snatch, 123, **123**
        jump shrug, 121, **121**
        jump squat, 117, **117**
        kettlebell alternating swing, 119, **119**
        kettlebell snatch, 120, **120**
        seated pause box jump, 118, **118**
    hip-dominant exercises, 159–65, **159–65**
        dumbbell one-leg Romanian deadlift, 162, **162**
        good morning, 160, **160**
        one-leg back extension, 161, **161**
        Romanian deadlift, 159, **159**
        seated good morning, 163, **163**
        stability ball leg curl, 164, **164**
        val slide leg curl, 165, **165**
    kettlebell Tabata exercise
        two-handed swing, 187, **187**
    knee-dominant exercises, 126–32, **126–32**
        back squat, 127, **127**
        Bulgarian split squat, 129, **129**
        drop lunge, 130, **130**
        front squat, 126, **126**
        overhead squat, 128, **128**
        single-leg squat, 131, **131**
        split squat, 132, **132**
    place in regular lifting schedule, 114
    rest intervals, 110–14
    upper body pull exercises, 142–50, **142–50**
        bent-over row, 148, **148**
        cable face pulls, 149, **149**
        chinups, 143, **143**
        horizontal pullups, 145, **145**
        one-arm dumbbell plank row, 150, **150**
        one-arm horizontal pullup, 147, **147**
        pullups, 142, **142**

Timed sets (cont.)
    upper body pull exercises (cont.)
        side-to-side pullups, 144, **144**
        suspended rows, 146, **146**
    upper body push exercises, 133–41, **133–41**
        bench press, 133, **133**
        dips, 140, **140**
        dumbbell alternating bench press, 135, **135**
        dumbbell half bench press, 136, **136**
        dumbbell push press, 139, **139**
        incline press, 134, **134**
        push jerk, 138, **138**
        push press, 137, **137**
        suspended pushup, 141, **141**
    using 30 seconds work: 30-second rest intervals, 10–
        11, <u>111</u>, 111–12, <u>170</u>, 170–71, **170–71**
        kettlebell front squat (one sided), 170, **170**
        kettlebell sumo jump squat, 171, **171**
    using 30 seconds work: 60-second rest intervals, 110,
        111, <u>166</u>, 166–69, **166–69**
        plank walkup, 167, **167**
        plank with weight transfer, 169, **169**
        reverse lunge, 166, **166**
        split squat jump, 168, **168**
    using 30 seconds work: 90-second rest intervals, 112–
        13, <u>113</u>
    using 40 seconds work: 20-second rest intervals, 112,
        <u>112</u>, <u>172</u>, 173–84, **173–84**, 173–86, **173–86**
        kettlebell alternating swing, 176, **176**
        kettlebell swing, 174, **174**
        medicine ball burpee, 186, **186**
        medicine ball overhead squat, 185, **185**
        medicine ball pushup, 183, **183**
        medicine ball split jump, 182, **182**
        medicine ball straight leg situp, 184, **184**
        TRX 180 degree jumps, 179, **179**
        TRX atomic pushup, 178, **178**
        TRX rows, 180, **180**
        TRX superman, 181, **181**
        val slide ab slide, 175, **175**
        val slide atomic pushup, 173, **173**
        val slide sled push, 177, **177**
        workout #1, 173–77, **173–77**
        workout #2, 178–81, **178–81**
        workout #3, 181–84, **181–84**
Tire flips, 211, **211**
Treadmill, <u>208</u>
TRX 180 degree jumps, 179, **179**
TRX atomic pushup, 178, **178**
TRX rows, 180, **180**
TRX superman, 181, **181**
TRX/suspended ring jump squats, 215, **215**
TRX/suspended ring mountain climbers, 214, **214**
24s, 10–11, 113, <u>113</u>
20/10s, <u>115</u>
Two-handed swing, 52, **52**, 60, **60**, 187, **187**, 188, **188**

U
Upper body pull exercises, 142–50, **142–50**
    bent-over row, 148, **148**
    cable face pulls, 149, **149**
    chinups, 143, **143**
    horizontal pullups, 145, **145**
    one-arm dumbbell plank row, 150, **150**
    one-arm horizontal pullup, 147, **147**
    pullups, 142, **142**
    side-to-side pullups, 144, **144**
    suspended rows, 146, **146**
Upper body push exercises, 133–41, **133–41**
    bench press, 133, **133**
    dips, 140, **140**
    dumbbell alternating bench press, 135, **135**
    dumbbell half bench press, 136, **136**
    dumbbell push press, 139, **139**
    incline press, 134, **134**
    push jerk, 138, **138**
    push press, 137, **137**
    suspended pushup, 141, **141**

V
Val slide ab slide, 175, **175**
Val slide atomic pushup, 173, **173**
Val slide leg curl, 165, **165**
Val slide sled push, 177, **177**

W
Walking, for cooldown, 15
Warmup
    complexes
        barbell warmup, <u>14</u>, 16–21, **16–21**
        body-weight warmup, <u>14</u>, 28–33, **28–33**
        description of, 13
        dumbbell warmup, <u>14</u>, 22–27, **22–27**
    dynamic, <u>14</u>, 34–40, **34–40**
    greasing the knees, 14
    length of, 13
    for sprint and agility training, 15
Weighted burpee, 85, **85**
Windmills, 73, **73**, 158, **158**
Woodchop, 91, **91**
Workout logs
    complexes
        advanced, <u>231–32</u>
        beginner, <u>227–28</u>
        intermediate, <u>229–30</u>
        sample, <u>226</u>
    density training, <u>233–35</u>
Workout shake, 221, 222, 223
Workouts, sample
    agility training, <u>205</u>
    sprint training, <u>203</u>
Work-to-rest ratios, in sprint training, <u>202</u>, 202–3